Farm Animal Health and Disease Control

Farm Animal Health and Disease Control

JOHN K. WINKLER, D.V.M.
Large Animal Surgery and Medicine
Auburn University, Auburn, AL

Second Edition

Lea & Febiger • 1982 • PHILADELPHIA

Lea & Febiger
600 Washington Square
Philadelphia, Pa. 19106
U.S.A.

Library of Congress Cataloging in Publication Data
Winkler, John K.
    Farm animal health and disease control.
    Rev ed. of: Farm animal health and disease
control/Joseph H. Galloway. 1972.
    Bibliography: p.
    Includes index.
    1. Veterinary medicine. I. Galloway, Joseph H.
Farm animal health and disease control. II. Title.
SF745.W58 1982   636.089   81-18656
ISBN 0-8121-0843-4   AACR2

First Edition 1972

Reprinted 1974

Published in Great Britain by Bailliere Tindall, London

Printed in the United States of America

Print Number: 3   2   1

Preface

This book is primarily the work of the late Joseph H. Galloway, B.V.Sc., M.R.C.V.S. At the time of publication of the first edition in 1972, he was Director of the Vivarium and Assistant Professor of Physiology and Biophysics, Georgetown University School of Medicine, Washington, D.C.

Dr. Galloway planned and wrote the first edition to fill a need for a text outlining the principles of preventive veterinary medicine and disease control for agricultural students. His work has justifiably been well received. Animal science is indebted to Dr. Galloway for his scholarly and practical effort to provide an understanding of the principles of maintaining the health of farm animals.

I have edited and revised Dr. Galloway's book with the same objective. The intervening years between the publication of the first edition and this edition have furnished the opportunity for increased knowledge of disease prevention and publication of pertinent texts, manuals, and other teaching aids. These developments, plus the influence of my experience teaching animal science students and participating in dairy herd disease prevention programs, have prompted extensive revision of the text as well as updating some of Dr. Galloway's work.

Management of livestock to maintain health can be accomplished by application of known principles and methods. Managers will apply principles they understand. I believe this text, supplemented by current literature, will aid an instructor to develop this understanding by animal science students.

This book is composed of eleven chapters. The first consists of general information about the nature of types of diseases, defense mechanisms of the individual, control methods, diagnosis or identification of diseases, use of sanitation procedures for control, use and limitations of drugs and therapy, and the agencies provided by government to help to control diseases.

Each of the next six chapters covers diseases causing signs of change to a specific system or body component. The diseases in these sections were selected to illustrate principles and different methods of control and to provide useful information to livestock producers. I have found that grouping diseases according to the system or areas involved provides the instructor with an opportunity to create student interest in learning basic anatomy and physiology in order to understand the disease process.

The eighth chapter contains information

about diseases not currently present in the United States. These diseases require rigid application of disease-control principles to keep them from affecting our livestock. Chapter 9 provides brief discussions of the effects of poisonous plants and other substances on the health of farm animals. Chapter 10 offers examples of control measures that can be applied to some common parasites. The final chapter is a discussion of three commonly occurring tumors.

I wish to proclaim my appreciation of the fine work by Dr. Galloway. Although never having had the privilege of meeting him, I have developed a profound respect and admiration for his abilities. I also gratefully acknowledge the help in the preparation of "Agencies of Disease Control," in Chapter 1, of Dr. Paul Schnurrenberger and Dr. Robert Sharman of the Auburn University School of Veterinary Medicine.

Auburn, Alabama

John K. Winkler, D.V.M.

Contents

CHAPTER 1

General Principles

This chapter is designed to provide an understanding of disease, the reasons for its control, mechanisms of defense against disease, and methods of control. The scope of the subjects in this chapter is too wide to allow sufficient depth of coverage in this text. The reader is encouraged to use such texts as those listed below for additional study.

RECOMMENDED READING

Blood, DC, Henderson, JA, and Radostits, OM: Veterinary Medicine: A Textbook of the Diseases of Cattle, Sheep, Pigs, and Horses. 5th Edition. Chap. 2. Philadelphia, Lea & Febiger, 1979.

Jones, LM, Booth, NH, and McDonald, LE: Veterinary Pharmacology and Therapeutics. 4th Edition. Sections 1, 2, 13, 15. Ames, IA, Iowa State University Press, 1965.

Kelly, WR: Veterinary Clinical Diagnosis. 2nd Edition. Philadelphia, Lea & Febiger, 1974.

Merchant, IA, and Packer, RA: Veterinary Bacteriology and Virology. 7th Edition. Chaps. 7–13. Ames, IA, Iowa State University Press, 1967.

Title 9. Animal and Plant Products. Code of Federal Regulations. United States Department of Agriculture.

Introduction

Extensive use of farm animals for food, fiber, transportation, and other by-products indicates that they are necessary and desirable for the well-being of the people of the world. The health of farm animals must be maintained to efficiently utilize the resources that sustain them; to provide food, fiber, and transportation needs; and to prevent diseases that can affect both animal and man.

At present, the United States produces a significant surplus of food in spite of an increased population. The world as a whole suffers from a food shortage. Large populations in developing countries are not receiving an adequate diet of animal protein. Most of the cereal grains produced in the United States are marketed as livestock and poultry feeds. Much of the land area of the United States is used to produce forage, which is valuable only when utilized by livestock. Efficient use of these resources—cereal grains and forage land—depends on capable livestock production management and a profitable livestock industry. Loss of livestock by disease not only wastes a national resource, but also becomes a critical and tragic waste to the world's population.

Some livestock diseases directly affect human health and are called zoonoses. Such diseases as tuberculosis, brucellosis, leptospirosis, anthrax, and rabies are transmissible between animals and man and continue to be a threat as well as a compromise to the production of food. Laws and regulations to protect public health have been effective in controlling and reducing the incidence of such diseases.

The ingenuity and vigor of the farmer in the United States and intensive, successful agricultural research are responsible for providing sufficient food for this country, as well as a surplus which helps to feed the rest of the world. The agricultural industry, like all other industries in a free enterprise system, will continue to excel in efficiency as long as it remains profitable to the people furnishing the capital and their talents. Loss because of disease, either by the death of an animal or by reducing the productivity of the animal, reduces or destroys the margin of profit. The death of an animal due to disease not only represents a capital loss for the value of the animal, but also represents a loss of the resources and feed that were used by the animal. Illness or debilitation of an animal produces a loss due to reduced productivity during recovery from the illness, as well as to the expense and time consumed for individual attention. Therefore, uncontrolled diseases make livestock production unprofitable. Prevention and control of diseases are necessary to maintain a strong, vigorous livestock industry.

The purpose of this text is to describe and explain the role of scientists, veterinarians, and farm managers in the control of disease of livestock. The text will also provide an understanding of different types of diseases, their causes, knowledge required to identify or diagnose diseases, specific measures taken to control diseases, and the role of treatment of sick

3

TABLE 1–1.   Glossary of Terms.

Abrasion—A spot rubbed bare of skin or mucous membrane; a scraping wound.
Acute—Having a short and relatively severe course; not chronic.
Antibody—A specific substance produced by and in an animal as a reaction to the presence of an antigen.
Antigen—Any substance that, when introduced into the blood or tissues, incites the formation of antibody.
Biologic vector—An arthropod vector in which the infecting organism develops or multiplies before becoming
    infective to the individual.
Carrier—An animal that harbors in its body the specific organisms of a disease without manifest signs and thus acts as a
    carrier or distributor of the infection.
Chronic—Continuous; not acute.
Contusion—A bruise; a superficial injury produced by impact without laceration.
Disease—Any departure from the state of health. Any alteration of structure or function.
Fomite—Any substance other than food that may harbor and transmit a contagium.
Host—Any animal or plant upon which another organism lives parasitically.
Infection—Invasion of the tissues of the body by pathogenic organisms in such a way that injury followed by reactive
    phenomena results.
Laceration—A wound made by tearing.
Mechanical vector—An arthropod vector that transmits an infective organism from one host to another but is not
    essential to the life cycle of the parasite.
Parasite—A plant or animal that lives on or within another living organism at whose expense it obtains some
    advantage without compensation.
Pathogen—Any disease-producing microorganism or material.
Sign—Objective evidence of disease.
Susceptible—An individual who is not immune to an infectious disease by either natural or artificial means.
Symptom—Subjective evidence of disease.
Toxin—Any poisonous substance of microbic, vegetable, or animal origin.
Trauma—A wound or injury.
Vector—A carrier, especially the animal (usually an arthropod) that transfers an infective agent from one host to
    another.
Virulence—The relative infectiousness of a microorganism or its ability to overcome the defenses of the host.

animals in controlling diseases. In addition, there are chapters describing livestock diseases that commonly occur in this country and some diseases that are foreign but remain a threat to our livestock unless kept under strict surveillance and control.

An attempt was made in the preparation of this book to make it unnecessary for the reader to constantly refer to a medical dictionary. Definitions are provided in Table 1–1 to facilitate understanding of the discussion of general principles.

TYPES OF DISEASES

Most people think that disease is caused by microorganisms, such as a bacteria, virus, or protozoa. Diseases caused by microorganisms are infectious diseases and do cause losses. However, disease can be defined as an alteration of structure or function. This definition broadens the scope of disease to include at least six major types. To appeal to student memoriza-

tion, someone listed them as Degenerative, Anomalous, Metabolic, Neoplastic, Infectious, and Traumatic (DAMN IT). All these types of diseases affect the productivity of livestock.

Degenerative diseases are those in which structure (bone, muscle, organs) is altered by age, senility, disuse, or biochemical changes. Function is altered as a result of changes in structure. An example of such a change is the atrophy or shrinking of a leg muscle caused by lack of use. Another example is the changes resulting from advanced age, such as impaired sight, hearing, or joint function. A common degenerative change in old cows is arthritis or joint inflammation of the vertebrae or hips. Degenerative changes may be subsequent to other types of disease, such as prolonged malnutrition. Degeneration of any body structure may weaken normal function, thereby predisposing the animal to infection by microorganisms.

Anomalous diseases are manifested by abnormal structure or functions present at birth. Extra digits, limbs, teats, or under-developed organs are considered anomalies. Such characteristics as dwarfism are considered anomalous. Some of these abnormalities are heritable or congenital.

Metabolic diseases include those caused by nutrition, toxins, or endocrine activity that alters normal metabolism. Such diseases as milk fever (hypocalcemia), grass tetany (hypomagnesemia), and ketosis are common metabolic diseases of cattle. Endocrine disturbances, such as hyperthyroidism, alter metabolism. Although not strictly classed as metabolic, the digestive diseases, such as rumen ulceration, displaced abomasum, and cecal dilatation, are related to nutrition. Loss of cattle from metabolic diseases is considered by some to be as great as loss from infectious diseases.

Neoplasms are abnormal growths resulting from a wild proliferation of cells. These cells grow at the expense of normal tissue and alter normal structure and function. Neoplastic disease (cancer) is not as common in farm animals as in pets or people. The reason for this lower occurrence is related to the shorter life span of a farm animal. However, several neoplastic diseases, such as lymphosarcoma of cattle, cancer eye of cattle, melanomas of horses, and various other tumors, do cause serious economic loss.

Infectious diseases are caused by microorganisms that invade the body and damage normal structure and function. A microorganism that has a harmful effect is called a pathogen. Many types of organisms have this capability, and each causes a wide range of changes to normal structures and body functions. Infectious diseases are particularly costly because they may be contagious and transmitted from animal to animal, thereby affecting large numbers. A virus, such as the hog cholera virus, could spread from one animal to affect a herd, then an adjacent herd, and then to all the hogs in an entire area. Epidemics (or preferably epizootics when referring to animals) are the result of wide-spread dissemination of such organisms. This class of disease is so insidious and causes such great losses that it is the primary concern of all disease control programs.

Trauma means violent mechanical injury. A broken bone, a torn muscle, a deep cut, a bruise, a burn, or a puncture wound are all examples of traumatic injury. The potential for traumatic injury to farm animals is high, and losses of such animals from trauma are increased because of the possibility of subsequent infection.

Changes in body structure or changes in the function of component parts, such as tissues (e.g., muscle), organs (e.g., liver), or systems (e.g., digestive), usually produce detectable signs. For example, a tumor (neoplasm) growing in the spinal canal produces pressures on a segment of the spinal cord, causing nerve damage and lack of control of a limb. A simple contusion or bruise to a muscle causes swelling, pain, and reduced use of the muscle and a noticeable limp when the animal walks. An infection by a respiratory virus causes coughing, rapid breathing, lacrimation, and fever. These signs are caused by the response to the disease and the process of repair.

Signs of disease may be obscure and may develop slowly, as happens with paratuberculosis of cattle, which is a chronic debilitating infectious disease. In other instances, the signs may develop rapidly with spectacular changes resulting in death, as happens when animals are poisoned by chemicals. Rapidly developing diseases with exaggerated signs are called acute. If the disease process involves the entire body or a major system, it is also termed systemic. Hog cholera, pneumonia of calves, and mastitis of cows have acute systemic forms.

Disease processes may also be confined to a local area on the body or in a particular organ and may cause little or no systemic effect. For example, an infection in one quarter of the mammary gland of a cow may cause slight or moderate swelling and some changes in the secretion of that quarter but does not cause other changes. This type of infection would be classified as a local infection. If this infection causes the quarter to be hot and painful, it is considered a local acute mastitis. If it persists over a long period of time without pain or acute swelling but with continued altered secretion as evidence of infection, it is considered a local chronic mastitis.

Response of tissues to disease may result in inflammation. Changes due to inflammation are characterized by some or all the ''cardinal signs of inflammation,'' which include heat, pain, swelling, redness, and loss of function. Consider a simple laceration of the skin. The repair process initiated by the laceration consists of hemorrhage and increased circulation in the area (redness and swelling), pain because of the swelling, heat because of in-

creased local cell metabolism, and impaired function because of the pain and swelling. When the wound caused by the laceration becomes infected with a pathogenic microorganism, tissue destrucion around the area and multiplication of the infecting organism result in more swelling and pain.

The outcome of the simple laceration described may be determined by the care or precautions taken to keep the wound clean and free of irritation and contaminating bacteria and by the resistance or defense mechanism of the animal. When the wound is kept free of infection, healing takes place and new tissue closes the wound with little or no change. However, if the wound becomes infected and the defense mechanism cannot contain the infection, the pathogenic organisms will enter the circulation and cause general signs of disease. One of the most common signs of a generalized infection is fever.

Body Defenses

The body of an animal is protected from diseases in many different ways. Skin and hair covering protect against traumatic injury from pressure, heat, and cold. The bony skeleton protects and shields the vital organs in the chest or thorax. Hoof walls or cornified foot pads cover points of heavy contact and wear. Lacrimal secretions wash away irritating substances from the eye. The skull or cranium and the vertebrae protect the brain and spinal cord. Pathogenic or disease-producing microorganisms are prevented from entering the body by the body covering of skin and hair and by a built-in system that destroys them when they do break through. Microorganisms can enter the body through the surface of the skin, the mouth, the nasal

passages, or any natural body opening. Even the lungs are protected by a specialized epithelial cell lining of the nasal passages, trachea, and bronchi.

If the protective shielding of the outer surface of the body is compromised by cuts or abrasions, pathogenic microorganisms can invade and multiply. Or, if the number and strength of the organisms are too great, the natural protection barriers are overcome. When this happens, other defense mechanisms are stimulated to action. White blood cells in circulating blood rush to the challenged area to engulf or phagocytize the invading organisms and to form a protective barrier to further invasion. Cells containing antibodies to the invading organism destroy or neutralize its effect. A normal, healthy animal can overcome challenges by many pathogens. A weak, debilitated, or stressed animal may not be able to resist the invasion.

The phenomena responsible for protection against infection is termed immunity. Immunology is a science with recent extensive research and newly understood principles. In general, immunity is classed as either passive or active. That is, the animal has either acquired antibodies from an outside source, such as colostrum from its dam or serum from another immune animal, for temporary *passive* protection or has *actively* developed antibodies of its own in response to the stimuli of exposure to specific diseases.

Contagious and infectious diseases are caused through the invasion of the body by microorganisms, which are single-celled creatures that multiply by the simple process of division; however, in adverse circumstances, some microorganisms may form spores, which are capable of withstanding conditions that would be fatal in the vegetative stage. Microorganisms range in structure and size from the invisible, or ultramicroscopic, viruses, to the simple bacteria seen through a microscope under fairly high magnification, to the more complex, comparatively large microorganisms, such as protozoa, which are visible under fairly low magnification. Many microorganisms elaborate toxins, the poisonous effect of which may damage the tissues, destroy the body defenses, and cause death.

The body is invaded most frequently through the natural orifices (the mouth, the nose, the genital organs) or through broken or damaged skin. Some disease agents gain admission through external vectors, such as ticks or biting flies. These vectors become infected when ingesting the blood of a diseased animal and transmit the microorganisms when they move to feed on another animal. The infective agent is introduced by the mouth parts of the insect. For a time after introduction, the microorganisms apparently have no harmful effect on their host, but they nevertheless multiply at as great a rate as allowed by the defensive mechanisms of the host. Their presence stimulates the host to produce antibodies to combat the microorganisms. The defense may be so effective that the invader is overcome immediately or, if not, is unable to multiply quickly enough to harm the host. In this instance, the animal may become a carrier.

With an effective defense, the animal is immune to a particular microorganism. A state of immunity may be characteristic of a breed, that is, genetic in nature, or more commonly, it may be the acquired protection afforded either by a reservoir of antibodies built up by a former invasion of the same type of microorganism or by the passive immunity provided by colostrum. If the infective agent is not checked, it may multiply within an organ or throughout the body and, ultimately, will give rise to the signs characterizing a specific disease. Signs are not present in the early, incubative stage, when the initial multiplication is proceeding. They appear after the microorganisms have overcome the body's defenses and are the signs of the damage done by the microorganisms.

The newborn animal receives many of the antibodies possessed by its dam in the colostrum so that it starts life protected to a certain extent against the common diseases in its environment. The newborn is soon exposed to a host of pathogenic microorganisms and, with the help conferred by its dam, overcomes the infection, if not too virulent, until it begins to make its own antibodies. Once the young animal's own protective mechanism begins to function, its immunity increases with each fresh exposure. In this respect, indigenous livestock are superior to livestock without the same disease experience. A slightly troublesome or even unimportant disease to the former may be fatal to the latter when first exposed to a contaminated farm or area. Thus, all new importations should be held in quarantine on the periphery of a farm or ranch until they have been gradually exposed to local conditions.

The ability of the body to react to invasion is the basis of the protection offered by vaccines and other biologic products. These products take one of several forms:

1. The infective agent is attenuated to such a state of impotence that, when injected into the body, it merely stimulates the tissues to react to produce antibodies.

2. The dead infective agent, or its modified toxins, in solution, provokes the body to produce antibodies or antitoxins.

3. Antibodies elaborated in the serum or colostrum of some animals are extracted for use in other animals.

An animal is encouraged by the first two products to develop its own protective mechanism and to *acquire* active immunity before danger arises. With the last product, the immunity of another is *passively* conferred upon the animal (Table 1–2). The *acquired* immunity needs time to develop so that it will be ready to counteract infection when it occurs. Attempts made to produce such immunity after infection has taken place are either without effect or possibly harmful. Once active immunity has been acquired, it remains effective for a considerable time, sometimes for life. The *passive* immunity, on the other hand, is conferred immediately by the introduction of antibodies into the body. This usefully augments the animal's own disease protection mechanism, and passive immunity can be successfully induced either im-

mediately before or after infection; it has no permanency and is lost comparatively quickly. A particular type of passive immunity is the immunity of the newborn acquired through intake of colostrum.

The outcome of infection depends on two factors: the invading microorganism and the animal host. The microorganism may be so virulent that death quickly follows infection, or it may be attenuated by unfavorable circumstances so that it loses its strength and is easily dealt with by the host. The virulence of the microorganism may be increased by animal passage to such an extent that it overpowers the host. On the other hand, however, it may be so attenuated by passage that signs are mild and easily overlooked.

Animals vary in relation to susceptibility. An animal may be so weakened by inadequate feeding, poor housing, overwork, or concurrent disease that an otherwise mild infection, thus facilitated, becomes disastrous. On the other hand, the vitality associated with proper management, good feeding, and the absence of stress may minimize either the infection or its effects. The natural defenses of the body are quickly brought into action, the antibodies are elaborated, and immunity is acquired.

Biologic products of one kind or another have been designed to give some degree of protection against many of the common contagious diseases. Some are more effective than others. Those used against the viral diseases are generally the most effica-

TABLE 1–2. Types of Immunity.

Immunity			
Passive		Active	
Naturally Acquired	Artificially Acquired	Naturally Acquired	Artificially Acquired
Breed resistance	Serum	Recovery from disease	Vaccines
Colostrum from dam	Gamma globulin	Subclinical infection while nursing on colostrum	Bacterins

cious, as is the immunity acquired against these diseases under natural conditions. The bacterial diseases can be countered by the same means, but the immunity resulting from the natural bacterial infection is often not strong or lasting; it has to be repeated periodically if immunity is to be maintained.

Years of research and testing have given us more and better biologic weapons against livestock diseases, but one feature about them has remained the same—they must be used with utmost care because they are made from disease-producing organisms or their products.

Precautions and guides for handling, storage, and use of veterinary biologicals licensed by the U.S. Department of Agriculture can be found on the label or container of the product. Success with these products hinges on properly timed and skillful administration of dosage prescribed for a specific disease. Failure to observe important precautions could endanger thousands of animals.

To help to assure that veterinary biologicals are safe and effective, the U.S. Department of Agriculture Biologics Division licenses manufacturers and evaluates biologicals for safety and potency. Products of approved manufacturers can be identified by the U.S. license number appearing on the label of each container.

Modern biologicals and good husbandry practices not only prevent heavy disease losses in individual herds or flocks but also help to stem widespread outbreaks of infectious or contagious disease. A veterinarian or livestock extension agent in a particular area can provide information about when to vaccinate and about the diseases from which livestock should be protected. Vaccines and other biologicals, however, should not be considered as substitutes for good sanitation, good feeding, and other management practices that promote good animal health.

It is poor management to wait until a disease has occurred before initiating a vaccination program. Animals need 1 to 2 weeks after vaccination to acquire active immunity. Since the occurrence of disease may vary by origin, by region, by year, and by season, it is wise to plan a program well in advance of the expected arrival of diseases in any area. Further, federal or state requirements for vaccination may have to be satisfied to carry out plans for marketing livestock.

VACCINES

Live Virus Vaccine

Live virus vaccine is produced by inoculation of live virus into a medium, such as chick embryo. The virus is permitted to grow, and the vaccine is prepared from the infected fluids and tissues of the embryo. Care should be used in the administration of live virus vaccine as the vaccine itself may serve as a means of spreading the disease to susceptible animals.

Modified Live Virus Vaccine

Modified live virus vaccine is prepared by processing the disease-causing virus in such a way that it no longer causes disease but stimulates immunity.

Desiccated Vaccine

Desiccated vaccine is freeze-dried vaccine that must be reconstituted to a liquid state before use by addition of a diluent, usually distilled water.

Monovalent Vaccine and Monovalent Bacterin

Monovalent vaccine and monovalent bacterin are biologic products used to stimulate immunity to a single-disease organism.

Polyvalent Vaccine and Polyvalent Bacterin

Polyvalent vaccine and polyvalent bacterin are biologic products that stimulate immunity to two or more disease organisms.

ANTISERUM

Antiserum is used for quick protection against a disease. It contains sufficient antibodies to provide protection for 2 to 4 weeks. More lasting immunity is obtained against some diseases by using a vaccine simultaneously with antiserum. Large doses of an antiserum may have some curative value and may be used in treating diseases refractory to other types of treatment.

ANTITOXIN

Antitoxin is injected to neutralize poisons or toxins caused by an invading disease microorganism and to produce short-lived immunity similar to that produced by antiserum. Antitoxins contain large numbers of antibodies.

BACTERIN

Bacterin is used to stimulate immunity against bacterial diseases. It contains a standardized number of killed bacteria. Upon injection, a bacterin causes an animal to produce antibodies that will fight future invasions of the same type of bacteria.

Mixed bacterin contains standardized numbers of four or more bacterial species and is used to prevent conditions attributable to the microorganisms used in making the product.

DIAGNOSTIC AGENTS

Diagnostic agents and diagnostic antigens are biologicals used to detect and diagnose disease, either by causing a typical reaction following injection into an animal (diagnostic agent) or by producing standards in laboratory blood tests (diagnostic antigen).

ADMINISTRATION OF BIOLOGICALS

Biologicals should be administered by a veterinarian whenever possible. Only a person with knowledge of animal diseases and experienced in the use of biologicals should attempt immunization of animals.

One inept in this procedure could endanger an entire herd.

Vaccinate only healthy animals. Immunization is adversely affected by anything that lowers resistance or causes stress to the animal. This includes overwork, exposure to cold, lack of proper feed, shipment over long distance (especially in cold and stormy weather), and chronic infections or presence of parasites. To increase chances for successful immunization, eliminate as many adverse conditions as possible, free animals of parasites, treat chronic respiratory infections, eliminate deficiencies in diets, and protect animals from cold and dampness.

Age is also a factor in immunization. Neither very young nor very old animals respond as well to vaccination as do those between these extremes. In the very young, a passive immunity should be employed because the antibody-producing system has not yet developed. In the very old, the antibody-producing system may be overworked, and therefore, a passive immunity is desired.

ROLE OF COLOSTRUM

Because all animals are highly susceptible to disease after birth, nature has provided a means of transmitting immunity from mother to offspring. This resistance is provided primarily by antibodies developed in the dam following exposure to infections. Newborn animals are born without protective antibodies, but they begin to be protected a few minutes after their first meal of colostrum. As the newborns grow, they develop their own protection and rely less on their mother's immunity.

Antibodies are concentrated primarily in the gamma globulin serum protein in the blood. Young animals are born with practically none of this vital protein. Gamma globulin of colostrum is absorbed intact by the cells lining the intestinal ract and is transferred immediately to the blood. Within minutes after nursing, antibodies are found in the blood. The cells continue to absorb whole particles of gamma globulin until they are completely filled with this protein. If gamma globulin is not present in sufficient quantities, other soluble proteins are absorbed in an apparent attempt to meet the emergency; if the cells become filled, they cannot use gamma globulin, which may become available later. Normally, during the first 24 hours a dam provides a quantity of colostrum gamma globulin equivalent to that contained in her entire circulation. Nearly one half of this quantity is secreted by the dam and ingested by the offspring during the first nursing period. The first colostrum has a protein content of 14 to 20% and is 5 to 6 times higher in gamma globulin than serum.

The absolute amount of gamma globulin absorbed by the various species is different; however, one half of the gamma globulin ingested during the first nursing period is found in the blood of the pig when peak levels are reached 6 to 12 hours later. At this time, gamma globulin levels are 2 to 3 levels higher than in adult hogs. After 24 to 48 hours, gamma globulin levels fall rapidly for 7 to 10 days, decrease more slowly for an additional 2 weeks, stabilize for 3 to 4 weeks, and then gradually rise. The same general pattern applies to all species of livestock.

At first glance it would appear that newborn animals are provided with an excess of antibodies contained in gamma globulin. Under ideal conditions, this is true. There is little need for production of antibodies, and all protein can be used for body building or growth. Ideally, between 1 and 2 weeks of age, the young animals begin to adjust to environmental disease agents and produce their own active antibodies for additional protection.

The longer the period following birth before a high gamma-globulin level is reached in the circulation of the newborn, the greater the chance for infection to become established. The antibody-producing mechanism of young animals is called on to produce excessive amounts of gamma-globulin in competition against protein for growth; thus, growth is reduced. This is always the case, even though disease may not be apparent.

Any condition that tends to decrease the colostrum flow of the dam immediately after birth has a detrimental and long-lasting effect on newborn animals. Such factors as difficult parturition, digestive upsets, metritis, and mastitis, are easily recognized. Mental anxiety or distress of the mother, a major, complicated, and frequently unrecognized problem, often is an underlying factor in any of these conditions.

Transmission of immunity from the dam to the newborn is a unique phenomenon without peer in the prevention of infectious diseases under the primitive, natural conditions in which it is involved. The frequency of infections in young animals, however, indicates that transmission of immunity does not prevent disease under ordinary management conditions. Therefore, the following suggestions are made in this light.

1. Expect dams to transfer only immunity that they possess. Even though a nursery area may look clean, it still represents a different environment from the gestation area and may harbor many agents from previous breeding periods in spite of conscientious sanitation.

2. Recognize that many chronic infections induce poor immuniy; therefore, little protection is transmitted to young animals. Eradication should be practiced where possible. Isolate young animals that become sick to prevent seeding to other young animals.

3. Practice recognized vaccination for disease that can be prevented, and thus maintain a high level of immunity by artificial means.

4. Handle dams as easily and quietly as possible prior to and at parturition. Parturition is surrounded by varying degrees of emotionalism in all species of animals.

5. Provide comfortable quarters in a draft-free, warm, protected area for all dams with newborns.

Disease Control Methods

After understanding what disease is and how it is recognized, the question of prevention or control must be examined. The assumption that all potential causes of disease can be removed is idealistic and impractical. This assumes a complete understanding of all diseases and the capability of removing the causes. Such sciences as microbiology, parasitology, and entomology deal with living organisms that cause infectious disease. Pathology is the science that deals with what disease does to an animal. These sciences, plus those dealing with normal structure and function, help to create an understanding of the causes. The capacity to remove the cause depends on knowledge of the requirements for sustaining living organisms, how they infect animals, and the effective means of destroying or neutralizing them. Removal of the causes of degenerative diseases requires an understanding of the function of all body systems, of cellular metabolism, and of the aging process. Causes for anomalies may be related to genetics or the effect of chemicals or infectious disease. Diseases of metabolism and nutrition require a knowledge of normal function and requirements to understand causes of change. Causes of traumatic disease are most obvious and easily understood. The removal of factors in the environment that are potential causes of traumatic disease is the easiest disease control method to accomplish, but is also the most neglected.

A major accomplishment in the prevention of infectious disease was proving that living organisms cause disease and that microorganisms always originate from some other organisms, be they plant or animal. In 1863, a French scientist demonstrated that anthrax organisms could be shown in the blood of sheep that died of anthrax disease and that the organisms would multiply if kept under suitable con-

ditions. Later, in 1876, the noted German bacteriologist, Koch, showed conclusively that the organisms demonstrated by the French scientist could be grown on artificial media and were, therefore, the cause of anthrax in animals and people. From the early work of Koch, scientists now know how to grow microorganisms, how to produce disease with them, and how to make them into protective vaccines. However, that was only the beginning of the programs to protect animals from transmissible diseases.

Research workers had to learn how to produce each disease they studied so that they could supply themselves with sick animals with which to work. This task in itself was tremendous. Some of the questions they sought were: How do microorganisms cause death? Where do they grow in sick animals? How do they escape from sick animals? How long will they live outside the animal's body? What substances will kill the microorganisms?

The bacteria causing brucellosis in cattle multiply in the pregnant uterus and in the udder. Brucella organisms escape with the calf at the time of birth, in the discharge from the uterus a few days or weeks after abortion or birth, and in the milk of the dam. Anthrax organisms from infected animals may escape in discharges from the nose, in the urine, and in feces. Anthrax spores can live for 50 years or more in soil, even when exposed to bright sunlight and dry air. Brucella organisms, on the other hand, are usually destroyed in a few days if exposed to direct sunlight or dry air.

Animals may appear healthy and yet can spread microorganisms causing such diseases as tuberculosis, brucellosis, glanders, and coccidiosis. This discovery clarified the disappointing results that had followed attempts to eradicate diseases from infected herds by removing all animals showing signs. The carrier animals were not removed, and they continued to spread infection.

Much work has been done to find methods of detecting carrier animals that exhibit no signs. Governmental agencies have been instrumental in developing reporting procedures that make it possible to control many diseases by preventing exposure. The basic principles concerned in accomplishing this task can be divided into two parts: (1) the diagnosis of an endemic infection, and (2) the prevention of direct or indirect contact between disease-free animals and infected animals, or contaminated premises, equipment, feed, or vehicles.

By a system of reporting, state and federal veterinarians in various parts of the country learn where infection may be endemic. This may be done by making careful and repeated examinations of suspected animals, by examining animals passing through public stockyards, by requiring health certificates for all animals moving through interstate transportation systems, and by requiring veterinarians in the field to make reports of important infectious and contagious diseases. When a particular infectious disease is reported, trained personnel examine the herds or flocks from which it has been reported to determine the extent of the disease, and, if necessary, to establish a quarantine. Sometimes, a combination of physical examination and diagnostic testing is the standard procedure. If suspicious cases are found, the veterinarian may collect material and send it to a laboratory for tests. Sometimes, however, signs and lesions are so typical that the diagnosis is made without laboratory confirmation. For some diseases, the veterinarian relies solely on diagnostic tests.

Preventing contact between diseased and healthy animals often is difficult. The easiest and most economical way to prevent contact is to separate all diseased and exposed animals from healthy animals.

The suspect animals are then given curative treatment and held in isolation until they are free of infection. At the same time, all contaminated premises are cleaned and disinfected. This procedure eradicates disease by destroying the infectious agent at its source. Leaving healthy animals in a contaminated area continues the possibility of infection and the spread of disease organisms into an otherwise clean and uncontaminated area. Therefore, apparently healthy animals *should* be removed from the contaminated area to a clean area and kept under observation. Depending on the type of disease, infected animals may be held in isolation and quarantined on the same premises with little danger. However, such procedures are sometimes unsafe; for instance, any attempt to hold animals infected with foot-and-mouth disease on premises with other susceptible animals would probably be disastrous.

Infected animals (including man) are sources of infections. They are always potentially dangerous. Slaughter of infected farm animals may be the best procedure for actually preventing exposure and spread of diseases that are so infectious and easily transmitted that it is impossible to prevent their spread between sick and healthy animals kept on the same premises. Slaughter is also the method of choice in handling chronic diseases from which animals do not recover. Some animals may live with these diseases for months or years, during which time they discharge large numbers of the organisms on the pastures or into barns.

Because of the danger of carrier animals, the procedure in the United States is to slaughter all animals infected with certain serious diseases, such as tuberculosis. The government usually pays indemnities for slaughtered animals if the owners agree to follow programs of disease prevention prescribed by state and federal offices of disease control.

The causative agents of some diseases can be found in all parts of the carcasses of animals that have died from those diseases. Therefore, carcasses should be disposed of as quickly and thoroughly as possible by burning, sterilizing with heat, or burying deeply to prevent feral animals from disturbing the carcasses and further spreading the disease.

Premises contaminated with the disease-producing agents are potentially dangerous. Thorough cleaning and disinfection of barns, stables, and sheds exposed to disease-producing agents are necessary. Contaminated pastures present special problems. Spores of anthrax or blackleg organisms may live indefinitely in the soil. Viruses, on the other hand, may disappear from pastures in a relatively short time. Eggs, larvae, and immature arthropod and nematode organisms may infest pastures for a number of years. The plowing of pastures increases the danger of spores coming to the surface but lessens the danger of parasitic infestations. Plowing decreases bacteria and viruses by exposing them to drying in direct sunlight.

Protection from exposure becomes increasingly easier as the amount of infection decreases. However, care should be taken to prevent unusual movement of animals from infected premises into premises clean and free from disease. The most common way to expose and infect animals in disease-free herds is to introduce infected animals into the healthy herds. If a farmer or rancher needs to add animals to a disease-free herd or flock, he should insist on official health certificates covering both the animals to be added and the herds from which they originate. The animals the farmer buys should not be exposed in transit to infected animals or to contaminated trucks, cars, or pens. Newly purchased animals should be held in separate quarters for 3 weeks or longer, as animals that appear healthy may be harboring an infectious or contagious disease; they may pass all diagnostic tests and still transmit the disease to other unexposed animals.

Increased resistance is becoming an increasingly important factor in preventing transmissible diseases. It should be possible to increase resistance to some diseases by selective breeding. However, breeding farm animals for disease resistance is a long-term, costly operation. By natural selection, several breeds in different parts of the world have become somewhat resistant to diseases endemic in those areas; likewise, economic as well as environmental methods may have played a part in this natural selection.

Vaccination is a practical method of protection against transmissible disease. Vaccines give good protection against many of the transmissible diseases of livestock and poultry. No vaccine is absolutely safe or completely effective all the time; however, the practical value of vaccines has been demonstrated in many millions of protected animals.

Some vaccines give immediate and long-lasting protection. Some give immediate but short-lived protection. Some do not give satisfactory protection until 10 to 20 days after they are used. Some vaccines protect against only one type of disease, whereas others are polyvalent and protect against closely related microorganisms that cause diseases with different manifestations.

The use of vaccines is the most effective method for protecting animals against acute infectious diseases when epizootics appear in countries with ineffective quarantine laws and few veterinarians or regulatory officials. Countries with stronger laws and control methods may attack such epizootics more vigorously with quarantine and eradication programs. However, the use of vaccines alone usually does not result in the complete eradication of disease. By the same token, the combination of quarantine and elimination of infected animals—to prevent exposure of disease-free animals—with vaccination has been successful in eliminating some diseases. This combination of eradicating infected animals and vaccinating susceptible exposed animals has brought about the elimination in the United States of several devastating diseases that are still prevalent in other countries of the world, e.g., foot-and-mouth disease, rinderpest, contagious bovine pleuropneumonia, Texas fever, glanders, and dourine.

Protection against transmissible diseases is as important to the livestock producer as are good breeding, good management, and good feeding practices. Accepted protective measures should be included in the day-to-day operation of the livestock farm. This is primarily the responsibility of the livestock producer. Veterinarians, livestock sanitary officials, and research workers involved in the area of animal diseases perform important functions in this area. However, the programs they recommend cannot succeed without the wholehearted cooperation of the producer in carrying out these procedures. The ultimate objective is complete freedom from the transmissible diseases by which herds and flocks may be destroyed.

Diagnosis of Diseases

A cow lies in the middle of the pasture after the herd has moved in to be milked. The owner looks closely at the cow and urges her to get up. She makes a feeble attempt to rise but is either unable or too depressed to try. Is the cow injured? Has she become intoxicated by something she ate? Does she have a severe systemic infection? Is there some functional change in her nervous system, digestive system, or urogenital system? The process of determining the nature of disease is diagnosis. Making a diagnosis is a systematic process of collecting all the facts and making an objective evaluation of them while considering all that is known about specific diseases and their signs.

Why make a diagnosis? In the example of the "downer" cow, a diagnosis is necessary for the protection of the rest of the herd. If the cause of her disease is available to the rest of the herd, it must be eliminated to prevent further loss. Of secondary importance is the correct approach to restoring the cow to health, which depends on determining the nature of the disease.

Most diagnosticians have learned not to jump to conclusions, even when apparently clear-cut signs point to specific diseases.

The chance for error from hasty and superficial evaluations is great. Facts to be evaluated are collected by questioning the owner and examining records, if available, regarding all the information about the health of the herd, current production, reproduction status, nutrition, previous sickness and treatment, vaccinations, recent actions and behavior, and signs the owner may have noticed. Then, a careful examination of the cow is made to collect signs of altered structure or function. This physical examination involves an appraisal of the overall appearance of the cow, her general condition, and mental attitude. It also includes the collection of indices to her general condition by determining the body temperature, respiratory rate and quality, and pulse rate and quality. Increase in body temperature or fever may be an indication of a systemic infection or may simply indicate high environmental temperature. Decrease in body temperature could indicate intoxication. An increase in respiration could indicate excitement, fever, lung infection, or anemia. Pulse condition and rate are affected by pain, fever, blood volume, and general circulatory changes. Absence of changes from the normal in any of these values is just as important as the presence of a change. The examination proceeds by evaluation of each system (i.e., circulatory, respiratory, digestive, nervous, musculo-skeletal, urogenital), separately or concurrently, in as much detail as necessary. By doing so, the diagnostician continues to collect facts as to what is normal and what is altered. If the exact disease is still questionable after a complete physical examination is made, it may be necessary to collect tissues, blood, secretions, or excretions for laboratory analysis. Other diagnostic tools, such as radiographs, may help but are inconvenient to use in an open pasture.

Once the diagnosis is made, the course of action selected to control or prevent the disease from affecting the rest of the herd and to treat the cow can be initiated. If the disease is metabolic, nutritional changes can be made. If the disease is infectious, steps must be taken to prevent the other cattle from contact. If the disease is intoxication, the source, plant or chemical, must be found and removed. If the disease is due to a tumor or individual anomaly, the herd is not threatened. If the disease is traumatic, the cause must be determined and eliminated.

The need for and benefit from diagnosis of a sick animal or animals in a herd are obvious. But, what if the cow in the example were already dead? The need to protect the herd is still present, perhaps even more urgently because the cause can kill. The diagnostic examination entails the same collection of facts, but in this instance, the facts are collected from the animal carcass by postmortem examination or necropsy. Signs of disease in a dead animal are not always conclusive and are sometimes reduced or obliterated by postmortem changes in the tissues. These changes begin immediately after death and increase with time, especially if the environmental temperature is high. However, a skilled pathologist can learn much from a carcass that is fresh or that has been kept cool to reduce postmortem changes.

Since farm animals are usually condensed into herds, the losses from disease can be rapid and severe unless immediate active steps are taken to remove or block the cause and protect susceptible animals. Losses can be reduced by making certain that no sick or dead animal is undiagnosed. Veterinarians are trained in the art of diagnosis. The objective of their education and experience is fundamentally to develop an understanding of the signs of disease and the effects of disease processes.

Sanitation Procedures

NATURAL AGENCIES

Protection against infectious animal diseases lies primarily in avoiding contact with the infected animal or with infected material. The best way to avoid contact is to keep stock segregated to the extent that they do not mix with other animals, share facilities of feeding and watering, or use ground or accommodations upon which infection may still linger. Such isolation can seldom be followed completely. Under the most careful management, occasions arise when a calculated risk must be taken; more often, a slip is made by the farmer or rancher, an employee, or some other person who does not heed signs and warnings. One of the most common mistakes is the introduction of new animals into a healthy herd without taking adequate quarantine precautions. Another common mistake is accepting, without quarantine, the return of an animal to the herd after it has been exposed to the chance of infection, e.g., through its presence at a market or fair or auction yard, its transport in a truck that has not been cleaned properly, or its presence in a cattle chute or crush or some other place where animals are congregated.

Because the possibilities of infection are seldom absent, management must be designed so that if disease is contracted it may be controlled with the least cost. For that purpose, the stock should be divided into as many independent units as is economically permissable, and crowding within the units should be avoided. Each unit should consist of animals of the same sex and same age group. Animals of varying age groups must not be mixed at any one place because a latent infection can be passed on to susceptible animals.

Effective protection against disease lies in timely vaccination when possible, local segregation, division of the stock into manageable units, adequate nutrition, proper housing, and efficient supervision. One of the first duties to the farmer or rancher, to himself and to his neighbors, is to detect immediately the abnormality in his animals as the first sign of disease appears and to understand the posibility of its contagious nature. Contagious diseases must be detected early. If local conditions cause an owner to suspect the presence of a disease, or if he finds his suspicions are justified, he should immediately seek the help of his veterinarian.

An infected animal is an incubator for the microorganisms of the disease it harbors and can pass them on to all susceptible animals. The healthy animals should, therefore, be removed from close proximity to the disease without delay. Usually, the sick are allowed to stay on the infected ground and the healthy are removed to uncontaminated areas. Such action is not always convenient if only one or a few

animals are sick, but if the premises are a source of infection, the obviously healthy must be removed. By moving the sick, one is only increasing the extent of the infected area. This rule may not be as important when a disease transmitted by an insect vector is suspected because removing the sick removes the reservoir from which the vector becomes infected and tends to increase the area over which the infective microorganisms may be transmitted.

The second important step is to segregate the apparently healthy animals that have been in contact with the sick and to keep them in quarantine over the maximum incubating period. Under certain circumstances, particularly when the disease is especially virulent, it may be expedient to slaughter the sick and, in the instance of contagious disease, those animals that have been in contact with them. However, it is advisable to do so only on the advice of a veterinarian. It is risky, and often dangerous, to try to hide the presence of contagious disease by slaughter and disposal of the carcasses.

Much can be done to stop spread of infection by using chemicals that kill microorganisms or their spores. Some chemicals are more potent against one class of microorganisms than others, and if proper use is to be made of such material, some judgment is required in the selection of the best chemical for any particular occasion. However, none is of much use if its application is not thorough. Chemicals should be particularly directed against known concentrations of microorganisms, that is, the blood from the carcass of an animal that has recently died, pus and vaginal discharges, or the feces of an animal suffering from dysentery or scours.

All disease-producing microorganisms are adversely affected, and most are quickly killed by direct exposure to strong sunlight and dry currents of hot air; on the other hand, moist, warm air may favor their multiplication. Infective material should therefore be exposed, when possible, to direct sunlight so that complete desiccation is facilitated. Other agencies of physical disinfection contributing to the destruction of microorganisms are heat, cold, desiccation, and agitation.

Sunlight is the most potent, and its powers of destruction are enormous. Its efficacy is entirely due to the ultraviolet range of the spectrum, and its greatest wavelengths are between 2800 and 2400 angstrom units. Unfortunately, these ultraviolet rays have little penetrating power; they cannot pass through glass or translucent sheets or through clouds and industrial haze. The value of sunlight in animal buildings is thus unreliable.

Desiccation from fresh air and wind contributes to the destruction of microorganisms, especially if they have become exposed by thorough cleaning of a building or agitation of the soil. High temperatures also accelerate the destruction of exposed microorganisms, but cold, particularly freezing, temperatures may actually preserve them.

Another process is antibiosis, during which many bacteria and fungi produce substances antagonistic to other microorganisms. Penicillin and streptomycin are agents of this nature and have well-known antibacterial action. In the soil, pathogenic microorganisms can be acted upon by antibiotics produced by nonpathogenic organisms normally inhabiting the soil. Warm, moist conditions assist the action of these saprophytic agents.

Fire is the most effective method of destroying microorganisms and the material they contaminate and should be the first choice as a disinfectant whenever practical. For ordinary farm disinfection, dry heat applied by any other means is not so reliable, merely because of the difficulty of application. Moist steam under pressure has been successfully used for many years in sterilization and disinfection. The most resistant disease-producing agents are the spores of anthrax, but even they can be killed if boiled or exposed to live steam for a sufficient length of time. The momentary application of boiling water is ineffective, but prolonged boiling of any contaminated article sterilizes it with certainty.

Dry heat is not as effective as moist heat and may be dangerous to wooden buildings if safety measures are not exercised. The thermal death time for the nonspore-forming bacteria ranges from a few hours at 116°F to 60 minutes at 140°F or 5 minutes at 158°F. The most susceptible bacterial spores will succumb, though some may be extremely resistant. For example, Bacillus anthracis may survive for 90 minutes at 320°F, and Clostridium tetani may survive for 15 minutes at 284°F. Some spores may even survive heating at 572°F for 10 minutes. The transitory heating from a flame thrower must therefore be at a high temperature to achieve disinfection. Likewise, under moist heat, Bacillus anthracis may survive for as long as 15 minutes, and clostridial spores for as long as 300 minutes, at 200°F. The uncertainty of steaming is thus apparent. Although steaming is clearly a useful cleansing agent, it cannot be considered a reliable disinfectant when used in buildings where the microorganisms may be protected in cracks and crevices. Steam is more useful on equipment, but its powers are greatly increased by incorporating a detergent and disinfectant with the steam or hot water. Again, the presence of organic matter interferes with disinfection by heat.

METHODS OF MANURE DISPOSAL

Any method of animal husbandry requiring that farm livestock live in close proximity to their own bodily excreta is dangerous and preconditioning to disease. Intestinal and urinary discharges of livestock are seldom devoid of disease-producing microorganisms. In areas where animals are crowded into poorly drained enclosures and where there is no sunshine to dry the excrement, feed and water facilities are often contaminated with fecal material. Such a practice is detrimental to the health of livestock and is considered as chronic mismanagement from the standpoint of disease prevention.

No single step is so important to the health of livestock, especially those kept in small, closed spaces, as is the frequent removal of excrement in the surrounding area. Greatest care should be given to the surroundings of those animals that naturally prefer to take their food from the ground, such as swine.

However, experience seems to indicate that, in the loose housing barn, in which manure is compacted by the trampling of the livestock, there are advantages that must be weighed against daily removal of the excreta. There seems to be foundation for the belief that, in these almost dry, compacted manures, heat production and chemical changes exert a deleterious action on the microorganisms contained in the droppings.

Storage and final disposal of liquid and solid manure are of considerable sanitary importance. These substances have a rich intermixture of parasites, their ova, and, at times, the specific microorganisms of many well-known diseases. These pathogenic invaders may live for a considerable length of time in unsanitary surroundings. When animals are kept continuously in contact with excreta under crowded conditions, they are exposed to unbroken life cycles of many generations of pathogenic microorganisms.

Older methods for the storage of manure required the use of pits or storage areas. Such areas were believed to be far enough away from buildings that the danger of contamination of the immediate surroundings of the animals were reduced to a minimum. Manure pits or sheds were floored to control seepage and covered and screened to keep the animals away and to control flies. A fly-proof enclosure around such pits or sheds was considered

important, although in some instances such sophisticated protection was impractical. Parasiticides were often sprayed on manure piles, but this procedure was not entirely satisfactory in controlling the development of fly larvae. Spraying also was questionable from the viewpoint of producing resistance in the developing larvae. When this resistance occurred, larvae developed into adult flies that were resistant to subsequent attacks by the chemical.

One of the most practical methods of assuring a degree of fly control was the rapid drying of fecal material so that the fly eggs would not develop into larvae, or maggots, and subsequently into adult flies.

In yards for animals kept under crowded conditions, hard surfacing, especially with concrete and with appropriate drainage, is undoubtedly a most sanitary method. First, the ground is sloped so that drainage is toward one side of the yard, where a tile drain is placed to conduct the fecal material and urine away from the animal enclosure into an irrigation ditch or other place of removal. The accumulated animal waste is carried either directly in irrigation water to adjacent fields or into a sewage lagoon where it is fermented in time, as in any sewage disposal plant (Fig. 1–1). Sewage lagoons have been developed and serve a useful purpose in preventing undue pollution of adjacent streams with raw feces and urine from large animal feedlots or even from small barns and enclosures or individual farms.

Recommended lagoon design is intended to provide for waste disposal at a minimal cost without creating health hazards or public nuisances, especially from objectionable odors. Research has shown that the worst odors emanate from confined animal enclosures, and the least objectionable come from enclosures with partially slotted floors over a channel flushed daily into a lagoon. Therefore, where animals are kept in close confinement, an auto-

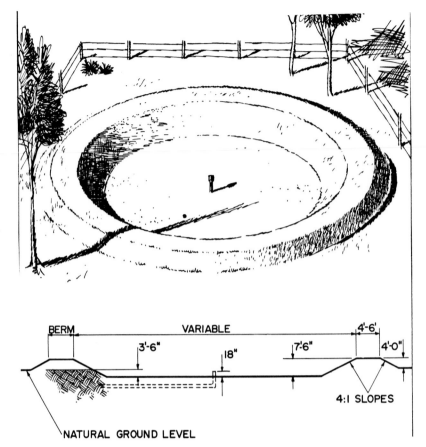

Fig. 1–1. Farm waste lagoon. (From National Hog Farmer Bulletin F19.)

matic flushing system under slotted floors, with drainage into a sewage lagoon, may be the most efficient waste disposal method.

The raising and feeding of livestock on raised floors, through which the manure falls, is not a new concept. Poultry have been raised on wire floors for many years, and in recent times, swine have been reared and fattened on slotted floors over storage pits, or pits that drain into lagoons.

The keeping of cattle on slotted floors has aroused some interest in this country. At least two steel fabricators offer eteel members for the construction of such floors, usually in conjunction with complete steel buildings (Fig. 1–2).

The interest in feeding cattle on concrete (Fig. 1–3) or slotted floors is an extension of the confinement feeding currently practiced; however, feeding on concrete floors has been done in parts of Europe for some time. The current interest in concrete or slotted floors is coupled with interest in

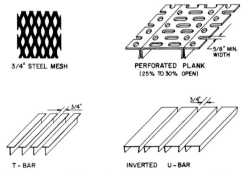

Fig. 1–2. Steel shapes for slotted floors. (From National Hog Farmer Bulletin F12.)

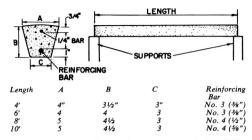

Length	A	B	C	Reinforcing Bar
4'	4"	3½"	3"	No. 3 (⅜")
6'	4	4	3	No. 3 (⅜")
8'	5	4½	3	No. 4 (½")
10'	5	4½	3	No. 4 (⅝")

Fig. 1–3. Concrete beam design. (From National Hog Farmer Bulletin F12.)

increased cattle density, as shown by recent experimental procedures.

Slotted floors appear to have some advantages over concrete floors because they are self-cleaning (the animals walk the manure through the slots). The manure forced through the slots may drop onto a floor for eventual mechanical cleaning or into storage pits from which it may be pumped by a sledge pump into a lagoon. This latter method appears to be the most desirable from the standpoint of flies and odor control. A properly maintained lagoon gives off little odor and does not provide a breeding place for flies. Animals tightly confined on concrete must be kept clean and probably should be bedded down in shavings, straw, or some other similar material.

One of the advantages of slotted floors or other means of intensive confinement is the ease with which they fit the idea of complete housing where climate dictates. The use of slotted floors is currently greatest in areas where climate control appears desirable, especially winter control.

Animals fed in close confinement are generally quiet and do not expend energy in play, as they do in traditional feedlots. Several investigations of the value of intensive confinement on both slotted and concrete floors under western conditions have favored the slotted floors. In eastern states, both sheep and swine are being reared on slotted floors with good results.

Slotted and concrete floors apparently have much to offer. However, as in other management innovations, patience is a

virtue and time spent on proper evaluation may be money saved. It is difficult to apply results achieved in other countries to local conditions. In the western part of the United States, concrete slabs elevated to provide drainage into irrigation ditches adequately meet local conditions. However, this sort of manure removal is of little value in those areas of the midwest and east where animals must be confined during the colder months of the year.

Because of increasing costs of commercial fertilizers, dairy farmers have returned to the practice of applying animal waste to the land. To avoid the cost of daily hauling and loss of fertilizer value caused by freezing, thawing, or washing, systems have been devised to store manure for application when fields are ready. Storage pits loaded from the bottom form a thick crust on the surface that seals in nutrients and cuts odor and fly problems. Another method is to scrape manure to a concrete ramp that slopes toward a storage pit adjacent to an irrigation lagoon. One side of the storage pit is a picket dam, which allows drainage of rain water or melted snow.

Sanitation is one of the most effective and still one of the cheapest ways to prevent disease. Disease is spread primarily in three ways: by physical contact, by contaminated feed and water, and by air movement. Physical contact is probably most important because it assures direct transfer of a virulent infective agent from one animal to another. Head-to-tail contact is important in the transmission of many infectious bacterial and viral diseases, as well as some of the parasitic diseases that gain entrance to the body through the digestive tract. Nose-to-nose contact transfers any pathogen capable of invading the body either through the lungs and respiratory tract or through the digestive tract. Body-to-body contact spreads external parasites and, occasionally, such skin diseases as ringworm.

Management stresses can be important when they involve comfort and sanitation.

Cattle and swine are expected to live and gain rapidly under many diverse conditions, which may vary widely from those under which they were raised. First, there is crowding. Instead of having acres per animal, as on the range, feeder cattle, swine, and lambs are crowded with many other animals into small areas. This crowding leads to the establishment of a social order—a graduation from the animal that always reaches the feed bunk or water trough first to the one that gets what is left after all the others have had their fill. The cleanliness of the bunks and troughs is also important; the cleaner they are, the more each animal will eat and drink to assure maximum growth.

Methods of manure disposal provide several advantages, both profitable for the producer and beneficial for the livestock. These are: (1) a saving in labor, (2) a possible increased production because of greater efficiency, (3) a practical solution to the problems of odor control and manure handling, (4) saving of bedding costs, (5) saving of feeding costs, (6) less chance for livestock to come into contact with pathogenic microorganisms.

STERILIZATION AND DISINFECTION

Most chemical disinfectants do all that is claimed for them by reliable manufacturers, but they must be applied as the manufacturers direct. Even the most efficient and effective chemical needs time to kill; the sprinkling of a disinfectant over a contaminated floor, for example, is generally futile, whereas soaking the floor with disinfectant could rightly be expected to be effective. Simple mechanical methods of cleaning, brushing, scraping, or flushing are often essential preliminaries to the application of disinfectant. Gross dirt cannot be treated effectively except by burning or deep burial.

Disinfection is generally effected by chemical agents. The lethal effects of disinfectants are due, in the main, to their ability to react with the protein and, in particular, the essential enzymes of microorganisms. Any agent that coagulates, precipitates, or otherwise denatures proteins acts as a general disinfectant. Among these agents are phenols, alcohols, acids, salts of heavy metals and hypochlorides, as well as heat in certain radiations.

Physical conditions, such as heat and radiation, and chemical substances that destroy microorganisms are the two broad groups of agencies used for sterilization or disinfection. The classical meanings of the words *disinfection* and *sterility* are still valid, but new terms have been introduced, and the old terms are sometimes used with modified meaning. Thus, the terms *antiseptic, disinfectant,* and *sterilant* are used for similar substances, and *disinfection* and *sterilization* for similar processes. The term *disinfectant* usually implies a germicide with little irritant effect on the tissues, whereas the term *sterilant* is coming into use possibly because *disinfectant* often implies a strong-smelling phenolic substance.

Sterility means *incapable of reproduction* or, in the hygienic sense, the complete absence of any form of life. The word is sometimes used more loosely to indicate absence of pathogens, ignoring the small number of harmless microorganisms that may not be destroyed. The word *sterility* should always be used in its strict sense.

In practice, the destruction of pathogens is often sufficient to control infection; the term *disinfection* is then used, particularly with reference to the surface of equipment, the interior of a room or building, or a large area. *Antisepsis* refers to the destruction of pathogens on the surface of a living organism or tissue.

A disinfectant is an agent that can destroy pathogens. It is usually a chemical agent. In the general context of disinfection, other terms are used that need accurate definition. A disinfectant is customarily applied to inanimate objects. In contrast, an antiseptic is an agent that eliminates infection on living tissues, but it may also sometimes be used to signify agents used in a weaker concentration than a disinfectant to render harmful microorganisms innocuous either by killing them or by preventing their growth. A sanitizer is an agent that reduces the number of contaminants to a level judged safe by public-health requirements. In disinfection, an absolute elimination of microorganisms is generally required; consequently, sanitizers are not effective. They are used, however, in the partial aerosol cleaning of the atmosphere in populated buildings, an increasingly common practice. A germicide is an agent that kills all microorganisms, and the term may therefore be considered synonymous with disinfectant.

The disinfection of a building can be accomplished by natural processes or by artificial means. Before discussing these in detail, it should be emphasized that cleaning is an essential preliminary to disinfection because organic matter considerably reduces the power of disinfectants.

Cleaning

Cleaning is of the greatest importance in all aspects of sterilization. Cleaning may be defined as the complete removal of all extraneous material, especially organic matter, that may harbor microorganisms. The modern fashion of chemical disinfection has tended to reduce the significance of cleaning. Heat may, in time, penetrate a film of dried organic material and kill microorganisms, but such a film may protect organisms indefinitely against all types of chemical sterilants or radiation. Aside from this, efficient cleaning removes about 99% of the bacteria on a filthy object and is, therefore, an integral part of the sterilizing processes. Organisms that survive are almost invariably spores or resistant cocci of no pathogenic importance. Spore-forming pathogens are the unfortunate excep-

tion, however. When destruction of these microorganisms becomes necessary, more drastic methods must be employed.

Factors Influencing Chemical Disinfectant Activity

Three basic phenomena are important for disinfection by chemical means: absorption of the compound by the cell wall; penetration into the cell cytoplasm; and reaction of the compound with one or more of the cell constituents. The properties of absorption and penetration in relation to the cell are not exclusive to the substance itself; they can be influenced by other constituents in the immediate environment, e.g., those affecting surface tensions and other physical-chemical properties. An example is the effect of aqueous solutions of phenol produced by sodium chloride, which enhances the activity of the phenol. The most important factor is, however, the chemical constitution of the disinfectant. Thus, the activities of alcohols and phenols in homologous series increase proportionately with their molecular weights to the limit of their solubilities.

Chemical disinfectants can more readily attack the cell of the aqueous phase natural to the organism. Conversely, any solvent that reduces the concentration of the disinfectant in the aqueous phase has the consequent effect of reducing the activity of the product. Oils, fats, and alcohols have this effect on phenol; its activity with these solvents is depressed. Emulsification of phenols in soap solutions appreciably enhances their activity. This characteristic is exploited in such preparations as Lysol and in various disinfectant fluids, which, for this reason, are more efficiently absorbed by the microorganism. Various inorganic salts also increase the power of disinfectants; for example, the absorption of phenol by the microorganism is greatly increased in this way.

The actions of osmosis and surface tension are also important. Some microorganisms are highly vulnerable to changes in tension. Reduction of surface tension generally increases the activity of a disinfectant; this is true with phenol, resorcinol, and hexoresorcinol, in which disinfecting ability is directly related to lowering of surface tension. The same is true with the quaternaries, in which cytolitic damage results in leakage of growth material from the cell.

Many disinfectants have a selective action for different microorganisms. Microorganisms respond to changes in pH value and, as every protein has its own characteristic isoelectric point, each responds individually and is influenced by the acidity or alkalinity of the disinfectant.

Complete disinfection is not an instantaneous matter; it takes place gradually. However, more microorganisms are killed at the beginning of the process than at the end. There is an initial lag period before activity commences. An examination of the number of microorganisms surviving at different stages during disinfection shows that the number of cells killed in unit time bears a constant relationship to the number of surviving microorganisms. Thus, after the lag phase, destruction of the cells is rapid at first but tends to slow up, so that eventual destruction of all microorganisms takes considerable time.

The activities of most disinfectants increase with temperature, but there are a few exceptions. The so-called temperature coefficient time is the measure of the change in velocity of disinfection per degree of rise in temperature. The coefficient is an exponential factor as well as a dilution coefficient. The effect of dilution, however, varies widely among disinfectants.

When disinfection is carried out on the farm, organic matter is almost invariably present. Organic matter always interferes with action of the disinfectant and may do so in the following ways:

1. The organic matter may protect the cell by forming a coating on it and preventing the ready access of the disinfectant.

2. The disinfectant may react chemically with the organic matter, resulting in a noneffective product.

3. The disinfectant may form an insoluble compound with the organic matter and destroy its potential activity.

4. Particulate and colloidal matter in suspension may absorb the disinfecting agent so that it is potentially removed from the solution.

5. Fats and oils may inactivate the disinfectant.

Bactericides and Bacteriostats

Generally, a bactericide kills bacteria, whereas a bacteriostat merely prevents growth or proliferation of bacteria. In general, the suffix -cide applies to any agent that kills microorganisms, whereas -stat applies to an agent that merely prevents their growth; thus, bacteriostat is a term that is occasionally used but has little relevance to the critical needs for sanitation. In practice, this distinction may be difficult to justify because vegetative cells of the bacteria that cannot grow usually die, although sometimes slowly. The difference in effect, therefore, may be a matter of time, concentration, and temperature. For practical purposes, we may assume that, if living cells cannot be recovered by cultural methods after removal of the chemical, the reaction is bactericidal. If living cells are recovered, then the action is bacteriostatic. It is often difficult to decide when a cell is dead, and this is only one of many reasons why laboratory tests may be unreliable as a guide to the efficiency of a germicide.

Most pathogenic microorganisms perish rapidly once outside the animal body, but unfortunately, enough may survive to cause renewed infection. Vegetative bacteria and viruses can live several months if protected with organic matter, whereas the spores of bacteria—for example, Clostridium tetani and Bacillus anthracis—can live almost indefinitely in the soil or in the cracks and crevices of buildings. Even the coccidial oocyst may survive for years in infected quarters.

Commonly Used Disinfectants

Hypochlorites

Chlorine or hypochlorite has many advantages. It is cheap, convenient to use, powerful, and has a wide antibacterial spectrum. Its greatest disadvantages are corrosiveness, strong odor, and neutralization by organic material. Corrosiveness may be minimized by using hypochlorite in cold solutions at a pH of 9 or higher; however, the solution becomes more bactericidal as the pH approaches the neutral point. Commercial preparations usually contain 9 to 12% and domestic preparations about 1% of the available chlorine.

Quaternary Ammonium Compounds

Next to hypochlorite, the quaternary ammonium compounds have hitherto been the most popular disinfectants. They are convenient to use, of low toxicity to animals, without appreciable odor or taste, and noncorrosive; but, they are relatively expensive. They are powerful agents against gram-positive organisms but are less efficient against gram-negative organisms. This is their greatest disadvantage. They are incompatible with soaps and ionic detergents, but can be used with alkalis and nonionic detergents. Alkalinity increases their bactericidal power, but they are weak detergents.

Working concentrations vary from 1:1000 to 1:20,000, according to the particular quaternary ammonium used, the temperature, the time, the alkalinity, and the percentage kill desired. Weight for weight, they are less effective than chlorine, but their other advantages far outweigh this fact.

Alkalis

Although generally regarded as detergents, caustic alkalis have a strong germicidal activity. Bactericidal activity falls rapidly with decreasing pH and is influenced by the nature of the anion. Hot caustic soda solutions at 1 to 3% are especially useful for killing spores—one of the main advantages of the use of alkalis.

Iodine

Although useful as an antiseptic, iodine has certain disadvantages as a sterilant. It has a powerful odor, stains badly, is not very soluble in water, and is expensive. It is readily soluble in iodide solutions and alcohol, but this method increases its cost and may produce a solution irritating to skin.

Iodophors

Iodophors are growing in popularity. They are prepared by the reaction of iodine on nonionic detergent in acid solution, and they have both detergent and sterilizing properties. It is claimed that the soluble iodine in this form has the same killing power as the available chlorine in hypochlorites.

Chloro-compounds

The usefulness of the chloro-phenols and related compounds has been established, but they are odorous and may be irritating. Chloramine-T does not suffer from these disadvantages, but is mild in action. Dichlorophene is more effective against gram-positive organisms and fungi than is hexachlorophene. Both have been popular as antiseptics. Hexachlorophene has a phenol coefficient of about 40 against Staphylococcus aureus and of about 15 against Salmonella typhi.

The Phenol Coefficient

The phenol coefficient of a disinfectant may be defined as the ratio of the killing power of the disinfectant to the killing power of pure phenol when determined under standard conditions. Obviously, the most important factors in such a determination are the conditions under which the test is made. The conditions under which phenol coefficients and other germicide tests are determined are given in publications by the U.S. Department of Agriculture.

Action of Chemical Disinfectants

Chemicals destroy microorganisms in a variety of ways. A few of the chemicals have only one type of action, whereas others bring about death by a number of different types of action.

Probably the most varied of any of the chemicals are the inorganic salts. Salts of various kinds in low concentrations stimulate the growth of bacteria and are important as buffers in growth media. In high concentrations, however, most salts are definitely toxic and hasten death. Salts vary in toxicity; sodium chloride is toxic only in high concentrations, whereas mercury bichloride is toxic in low concentrations. The toxic action of many salts, as well as other types of disinfectants, may be increased by the addition of sodium chloride. This increase is caused by increased dissociation and dispersion of the disinfectant, resulting in an increased effect on bacterial cells. However, the addition of sodium chloride to mercuric chloride lowers the toxicity of the latter.

Salts do not produce bacterial death by osmotic effects. Bacteria are resistant to changes in osmotic pressure and can live in distilled water as well as in rather high salt concentration. Salts do, however, exert a dehydrating effect on the media in which bacteria grow and thereby cause inhibition of growth and eventual death. Because of the dissociation of salts, most of the germicidal action is caused by the effect of ions on the bacterial cell. This effect may be the result of the influence upon cell permeability, the lyotropic action upon cell protoplasm altering cell metabolism, and the inactivation of enzymes on which the cells depend for the synthesis of food substance.

Oxidation is one of the most common methods by which chemicals cause death. Many salts, e.g., potassium permanganate and sodium perborate, are active oxidizing agents. The halogen compounds also are noted for this kind of chemical action.

Some chemicals used in sterilization are active reducing compounds. These, however, are not as commonly used as the oxidizing agents. The ferrous salts, sulfites, and thiosulfites are good examples of reducing compounds.

Many of the most effective chemicals form irreversible compounds with bacterial protoplasm by the coagulation of the protein. The salts of the heavy metals (silver, mercury, zinc, copper, and bismuth) are active in this manner. The derivatives of benzene, or the coal tar products (chief among which are phenol and cresol), are used widely as the basis of many commercial disinfectants. These chemicals in their purest state, saponified or altered by the replacement of a hydrogen atom by another chemical, cause the death of bacteria by the coagulation of bacterial protein.

Miscellaneous Compounds

Alcohol, especially ethyl alcohol, is considered by many to be a most effective antiseptic and is credited by some as a disinfectant. The efficacy of alcohol depends on the concentration. Investigation and experience have shown that 70% alcohol is most efficient; concentrations above and below that level are ineffective. Alcohols in general are more bactericidal in the higher molecular weights. They are expensive and, thus, used less widely than other substances.

Isopropyl alcohol is a more effective germicide than the more commonly used ethyl alcohol. It is used in the 98 to 99% pure state and is noncorrosive to instruments. The pungent odor of this alcohol is objectionable, and for that reason, it is not widely used.

Formaldehyde gained great popularity as a disinfectant in the days when infected dwellings were fumigated. Its value as a disinfectant in that procedure was due to its solubility in water; it is usually sold commercially as formalin, an aqueous alcoholic solution containing approximately 40% formaldehyde. Formalin is an effective germicide and is used not only for killing of animal and human pathogenic bacteria but also for treating seeds against fungi. This chemical is used as an attenuating agent for bacteria, toxins, and viruses that are to be used as immunizing agents.

Potassium permanganate was formerly used extensively in veterinary medicine as an antiseptic in drinking water for poultry, for which it seemed to have definite value. Potassium permanganate has also been used as a wound dressing and as a footbath for livestock. The stain produced by the chemical has limited its general use as an antiseptic, however. Hydrogen peroxide is not employed extensively as a disinfectant because it easily combines with organic matter. It does have some value as a cleansing agent for deep wounds, but its effervescent action belies its real value, and it should not be depended on to any great extent.

Investigations of the synthetic soaps or detergents have revealed that they have germicidal activity. Such compounds are classified as either cationic or anionic. The cationic detergents have greater germicidal activity than do the anionic compounds. Cationic detergents are active in the alkaline range, whereas the anionic detergents are active in the acid range. Most are nontoxic to living tissues and are safe to use as skin disinfectants. Some have been given internally to experimental animals without toxic effect, and benzalkonium (Zephiran)

has been shown to be an active germicide in a dilution of 1 to 80,000.

Desirable Properties of a Disinfectant

There are many disinfecting agents with variable properties. However, several properties should be found in any desirable disinfectant. Criteria for selecting an appropriate and effective agent for disinfection are as follows:

1. The disinfecting agent must be free of strong and objectionable odors.

2. The disinfecting agent must not be destructive to materials; that is, it should not be corrosive to the material to which it is designed to disinfect, nor should it bring about any other type of destruction.

3. A disinfectant should not remain strongly poisonous for a long time after its application. Some agents require a long period of time to become completely effective; however, the poisonous properties should not remain long after application or they themselves may cause poisoning to livestock.

4. A desirable disinfectant must not combine chemically with other chemicals so as to become inert.

5. An effective and desirable disinfectant must not be excessively irritating or poisonous when inhaled, as such a property would be undesirable from the public-health point of view.

6. A desirable disinfectant must be effective at ordinary temperatures, although warming a solution or warming the surface on which the disinfectant is to be applied enhances its killing power. Conversely, cold reduces killing power. Therefore, the desirable disinfectant must be effective at ordinary temperatures.

7. The disinfectant must be effective when diluted with water and must readily and uniformly mix with water because it is the universal solvent. A disinfectant that does not mix with water may cause several problems.

8. The disinfectant must be in such a concentration and in such a form that it may be readily and economically transported. The best disinfectant in the world would not be efficient or feasible if it could not be transported easily and economically to the place where it is to be used.

9. The disinfectant must be priced reasonably.

The foregoing has dealt with chemical disinfection and the ways in which it is brought about. There are also nonchemical means of disinfection. Mechanical agencies, such as cleaning and scrubbing, and the physical removal of organic matter are means of nonchemical disinfection. There are also natural agencies of nonchemical disinfection, including sunlight, heat, filtration, sedimentation, and time.

The USDA, in the interests of serving the public, publishes an official list containing those cresylic disinfectants permitted for use on equipment and animal quarters. All federal employees supervising the disinfection of infected or exposed cars, trucks, boats, other vehicles, stockyard pens, chutes, alleys, and premises are required to use a product permitted for that use under federal regulations. The current permitted list of cresylic disinfectants appears in Table 1–3. (All disinfectants are to be diluted in the proportions of 4 ounces to 1 gallon of water.)

TABLE 1-3.   Cresylic Disinfectants.

Trade Names	USDA Reg. No.
ARCO 50% Cresylic Solution	1516-13
B & B Cresco 16-N	6899-6
Bio-Lene Cresylic Disinfectant	5185-3
Bourbon Cresylic Disinfectant	1127-11
C-4 Brand Soluble Cresylic Disinfectant	363-25
Cento Discresol	1537-52
Co-op Cresylic Disinfectant	1222-13
Cooper Kerol	59-150
Cooper Saponified Cresylic Solution	59-7
Cres-A-Check	5884-7
Cresolutol	2617-31
Crestall Fluid	
Cresyline Cresylic Compound	551-177
Crystal Cresylic Disinfectant	888-5
Curts Cresylic Compound	1516-13
Diamond H. Cresyl Fluid	619-14
Franklin Cresolis	410-17
Germo Cresolis	784-17
GS Cresylic Disinfectant	10304-1
HVL Cresylic Disinfectant	10304-1
Hy-Kresol	670-19
Imco Brand Technical Cresol Compound	188-11
Jen-Sal Cresylic Disinfectant	411-32
Kremulso	148-56
Miller Cresylic Disinfectant	450-51
New M.F.A. 50% Cresylic Disinfectant	746-38
Palmer's Technical Cresol Compound	4821-4
Pfizer 50% Cresylic Disinfectant	1007-42
Purina Cre-So-Fec	602-19
Sanfax C-61	3635-48
S.O. Super Germite	522-14
Tekresol	984-3
U.C. Cresolis	623-8
Val-A-Saponified Cresylic Solution	189-11
Varco 50% Cresylic Solution	421-8
Varco Liquor Cresolis Saponatus NF XII	421-5
Warlasco 50% Cresylic	1616-38
Worrell's Crespolin	784-17

Use of Drugs and Therapy to Control Disease

Sick animals in a herd are an expensive nuisance and also may harbor, grow, and shed organisms dangerous to the healthy animals. The obvious solution is to isolate them, get them well, or get rid of them. Getting rid of them while they are sick may be possible by unloading them on an unsuspecting buyer. However, this not only may be illegal but also increases the possibilities of spreading and perpetuating

a disease problem. Getting rid of sick animals by extermination and burial may be practical in some instances, but it eliminates the possibility of recovering costs and potential value. If there is an economical cure for whatever affects the sick animal, it is usually feasible to attempt to restore the animal to health.

The decision to try to restore health must be based upon the hazards and costs of maintaining and treating a sick animal and the potential recovery and future value of the animal (prognosis). To know the hazards, costs, potential recovery, and value, one must know what is causing the disease and the nature of its course (diagnosis).

Treatment or therapy to restore health is directed toward aiding the natural repair process to return the animal to normal function or structure. Treatment may be undertaken by using medicines or drugs, by surgical intervention, or by time and nursing. Frequently, the best method for restoration is patient nursing without any interference with the healing process except through enforced rest in a comfortable environment. The livestock producer is not usually inclined to be patient in dealing with sick animals. Furthermore, his operation is tightly geared for maximum efficiency of production of healthy animals. The provision of extra labor and facilities for a sick bay or a hospital is not always feasible, and consequently, there is a strong tendency to seek a quick effective cure by a medicine or drug. In instances when large numbers of animals are sick, this procedure must necessarily be adaptable to the facilities and means of handling them. The use of expensive means of therapy, such as surgical intervention or long-term nursing and convalescence, must be evaluated in relation to the value of the individual animal and the facilities available. The use of medication, especially to suppress or cure infectious diseases, is frequently necessary as well as economically feasible.

Curing animals of infectious contagious diseases not only restores them to an economic value but also removes the threat of further spreading of the disease. Therefore, therapy or treatment does have an important role in animal disease control.

Because man has searched since the beginning of time for a means of relieving pain and restoring health, drugs or cures are abundant. Some are based on scientific proof of efficacy; some are simply time-honored, "known-effective" cures. There is a strong effort by the federal government to reduce the marketing of drugs without proof of efficacy. This effort has made the introduction of new products costly and time consuming and has caused the withdrawal of many products that were previously available. There are medicines or drugs for all purposes. Drugs can substitute for the function of organs, drugs can stimulate functions, drugs can slow down the actions or movement of structures, drugs can speed up movement, drugs can cause contraction or expansion, drugs can dilate and contract blood vessels, drugs can reduce pain, drugs can create euphoria or a sense of well-being, and so on. Some drugs can also stimulate body defenses against infection by microorganisms and some drugs can directly destroy bacteria. All drugs, if properly used, are directed toward speeding the recovery from disease.

However, because these agents are added to nature's effort to heal, they may cause damage (side effects) and they may remain in the body as a residue. Because the main purpose of farm animals is the production of food for human consumption, these residues of drugs are potentially a part of the human diet. Investigations have indicated that residues in meat, milk, or animal products are harmful to people if consumed. As testing techniques become more sensitive and as knowledge of harmful effects increases, more and more restrictions are being placed on the use of drugs for food-producing animals. Regulations for withdrawal time of drugs before marketing meat or milk are stringent.

The antibiotics are most commonly used for livestock to control or cure infectious diseases. Antibiotics reduce the number of microorganisms (primarily bacteria) responsible for infections. Some antibiotics are effective against certain bacteria and ineffective against others. None is directly effective against viruses and some actually help to stimulate the growth of some types of bacteria. Some antibiotics can be given to animals either orally or by injection. Some can be given only by injection. When some antibiotics are given orally to ruminants, their effect is either harmful or nonexistent. Some antibiotics can be effective when added to feed or drinking water. All antibiotics have definite characteristics as to what type of organism they affect, how much is required to be effective, how they are eliminated from the body, and how long and where they remain in body tissues. Present regulations require that no residues of antibiotics can appear in meat or milk sold for human consumption.

Antibiotics are effective not only for restoring health but also for preventing infections. Extensive unnecessary use of antibiotics as a substitute for other management practices is unwarranted and unproductive. However, they may be indicated as a means of precautionary support to stressed animals, e.g., after shipping. They are also indicated as support to an animal suffering from a viral infection to avoid a secondary bacterial infection. Their use as routine additions to feeds for growth stimulation or disease prevention is controversial and is considered by many to be a poor substitute for good husbandry.

The introduction of medicines to an animal's body can aid in restoring normal function. However, the indiscriminate use and overuse of medicines may delay healing and can actually cause further damage to normal functions. In the subsequent chapters describing specific diseases, emphasis is placed on means of prevention. In addition, if economical, effective, therapeutic measures can contribute to disease control, they will be indicated. Specific dosages and techniques may not be given because the rapidly increasing knowledge of pharmacokinetics is continually altering the concept of drug administration. The purpose of this text is to increase the understanding of disease control and the understanding of the limitations of therapy.

Agencies of Disease Control

The livestock industry of the United States is relatively efficient compared to that in many areas of the world. State and federal measures have been developed to combat diseases, but economic losses still occur. The greatest losses result not from death of animals but from the loss of meat, milk, or fiber when animals become debilitated.

As animal populations increase, the standards of management must also increase; otherwise, the ravages of diseases will be frequent and costly. Prevention of the spread of disease must be a consequence of cooperative efforts among livestock producers, state and federal agents, and veterinarians.

ACCREDITED VETERINARIANS

For many years, federal regulatory agencies have relied on the ability and the integrity of accredited veterinarians in the cooperative control and eradication of livestock diseases. Accredited veterinarians are practitioners who have been examined and certified as to their competence. They are privileged to cooperate with regulatory disease control programs that not only protect the livestock industry of the nation but also add to the well-being of mankind. Therefore, the accredited veterinarian is the first bulwark in the line of defense against ever-present animal disease.

Most veterinarians in large-animal practice are accredited by state and federal agencies to participate in activities that have a direct relationship to the economic diseases prevalent within a given area. The accredited veterinarian is obligated to report to the state and federal officials any outbreak, or any case diagnosed by him, of any of the reportable diseases and to seek additional aid and laboratory diagnosis to confirm the presence of the disease.

The veterinarian serves such programs as those designed for the eradication of tuberculosis, brucellosis, and scabies, and any other programs determined to be of economic importance. Thus, the local accredited veterinarian serves a multiple role while serving as a practitioner:

1. He is the regulatory official responsible for the testing, vaccination, quarantine, and disposal of reactor animals of economic importance.

2. He serves the public in such programs as rabies vaccination and the eradication of economic diseases.

3. He may serve in a public-health capacity by inspecting meat and milk and by supervising animal activities—primarily the movement of livestock—that have a bearing on human health.

The accredited veterinarian is responsible for the examination of livestock and the issuance of health certificates when livestock are moved across boundaries of states or counties—anywhere that cattle or hogs enter into interstate commerce.

County, district, or area veterinary services. In highly developed counties in many areas of the United States, the state, federal, and county veterinary organizations participate in activities of economic importance to livestock producers and are associated with programs aimed at preventing communicable diseases from spreading and from being transmitted to human beings.

State veterinarians. The office of state veterinarian has been created in each state for the purpose of controlling communicable diseases of economic importance within that state. The state veterinarian is the senior veterinary official within the state and is responsible to the governor, to the Livestock Disease Commission, to the Livestock Sanitary Board, or to the State Department of Agriculture, depending on the administrative structure of the state.

The state veterinarian evaluates the disease probabilities within a state, establishes livestock disease controls, and enforces those controls through regulations to prevent the widespread dissemination of diseases of economic importance to livestock producers. Whenever necessary, the state veterinarian may establish quarantines of a particular farm, an area, or an entire state. He establishes rules and regulations concerning the importation of animals from other states and approves the conditions of shipment into his state; the state veterinarian of one state may place a restriction on all animals emanating from any other state where a serious communicable disease may be present. He may serve at the head of the Veterinary Examining Board of the state, or may be an ex-officio member of the Board. He is responsible for the initiation of legislation concerning livestock disease control and serves as a consultant to the legislature in this area. He investigates violations of disease control regulations, cooperates with federal officials in the approval of accredited veterinarians, examines any cases in which violations of accreditation standards are suspected, and acts when the rules and regulations concerning eradication practices have been violated. The state veterinarian is responsible for the establishment of diagnostic laboratories to investigate and confirm the diagnoses of diseases referred by local veterinarians in the field.

FEDERAL REGULATORY AGENCIES

Veterinary Services, Animal and Plant Health Inspection Service of the United States Department of Agriculture is responsible, at the federal level, for the formulation and administration of cooperative federal-state programs for the control and eradication of animal diseases.

The responsibility for protecting the health of the nation's livestock includes full-scale or limited eradication programs; epidemiologic, laboratory, and field diagnostic services; and a continuing interest in all animal diseases, domestic or foreign, that are threats to livestock. To safeguard livestock producers in the United States from losses resulting from animal diseases, every possible effort must be made to prevent the introduction of foreign animal diseases, to stamp out promptly any infection that may gain a foothold, and to employ any adequate and established measures to this end. If the microorganism of any disease normally nonexistent in this country is introduced and threatens the livestock industry, the Secretary of Agriculture has the authority to cooperate with the states concerned in drastic eradication measures, including the purchase and destruction of diseased or exposed animals and contaminated material.

Among the regulatory features of material assistance in combating animal diseases are federal and state quarantines; campaigns for disease control and eradication; record keeping to disclose the extent and distribution of various diseases; stockyard inspection; testing of livestock before interstate shipment; cleaning and disinfecting of premises and vehicles; dipping of cattle and sheep for scabies; and the enforcement of the so-called "28-hour law." (This law prohibits railroads or other common carriers confining cattle, sheep, swine, or other animals shipped across state lines, for longer than 28 hours without unloading into properly equipped pens for feed, water, and rest, for a period of 5 hours.) Supervision over the production of biologic products and control of drug remedies are also important phases of the work.

In combating most infectious diseases of livestock, control of the movement of the diseased and exposed animals is essential.

Such control can seldom be accomplished without some kind of quarantine. The principal purpose for the establishment of quarantine is to confine the infection to the smallest possible area and to hold it there until it can be eradicated through the use of appropriate measures.

Several of the most serious communicable diseases of animals have not gained a permanent foothold in this country primarily because of the efforts of regulatory veterinary officials at ports of embarkation.

When an outbreak of a serious disease occurs, both federal and state officials impose drastic quarantine measures. To be effective and to have the support of interested agencies and livestock producers, quarantines must be appropriate for the particular disease being combated. These procedures may range from complete prohibition against the movement of all animals, produce, and vehicles (and even restrictions on human beings) to physical examination and movement under proper certification or official permit. Animals are subjected to prescribed observations and treatment before being allowed to enter into interstate commerce.

Although complete eradication is the final objective of all campaigns, two quite different principles, calling for correspondingly different methods of procedure, are involved. Diseases caused by or transmitted by external parasites may be effectively controlled by treatment of the affected animals for the destruction of the parasites or by eradication of the vector per se. On the other hand, bacterial or viral diseases are determined by diagnostic tests, and animals found to be infected are appraised and slaughtered. Owners of destroyed animals are indemnified by the state and federal governments within certain regulatory limits. Efforts toward the control and eradication of communicable animal diseases within the states are primarily the function of the respective state authorities; the direct authority of the federal government extends only to the control of the interstate movement of livestock from districts where disease is known to prevail. Authority to enforce local quarantines and to compel the destruction or the treatment of infected or exposed animals rests entirely with the states; consequently, the work of federal and state cooperative projects is done chiefly under state laws and regulations. State authorities attempt to proceed in harmony with the policies and practices agreed on by federal and state veterinary regulatory officials.

Infected animals are the source of all infection. They are always potentially dangerous. Therefore, slaughter of infected animals is usually the best procedure for actually preventing exposure and spread of easily transmitted diseases, such as foot-and-mouth disease. This affliction is so infectious that preventing its spread is almost impossible if sick and healthy animals are kept on the same premises.

PHILOSOPHY OF VETERINARY SERVICES, ANIMAL AND PLANT HEALTH INSPECTION SERVICE

The best economic treatment of livestock or poultry diseases is eradication. Preventing the introduction of foreign animal diseases and eradicating domestic diseases of major economic significance will ultimately eliminate the need for a continuous control program and its associated annual cost.

Veterinary Services, Animal and Plant Health Inspection Service

1. conducts nationwide state-federal cooperative programs for control and eradication of animal diseases.

2. suppresses the spread of disease through control of interstate and international movement of livestock.

3. is aware of the national and international disease situation and maintains the capability of dealing with foreign animal diseases.

4. administers laws to insure humane treatment of transported livestock and certain laboratory animals. Has responsibility for the enforcement of the law prohibiting the soring of horses.

5. collects and disseminates information on disease morbidity and mortality throughout the country.

6. provides for increased technical, managerial, and professional competence through continuous employee development and training.

APHIS is organized so that the deputy administrator has a group of regional directors under his control, one for each of the five major districts of the United States and two national animal diagnostic laboratories. Therefore, each state belongs to a larger district. Within most states is a federal veterinarian-in-charge, who is responsible for VS, APHIS programs. Under the veterinarian-in-charge for each state, variable numbers of veterinarians are designated as veterinary medical officers. They are responsible for all veterinary services programs and for the accredited veterinarians in private practice within the particular area, as their activities relate to federal and state diagnostic and regulatory activities. The activities of the veterinary medical officers are directly related to the activities on the farms and ranches; they assist the accredited veterinarians in diagnosis and issue local quarantines where diseases of economic importance are located. If a reportable communicable disease is suspected, they are responsible for soliciting the aid of local, state, or federal animal disease diagnostic laboratories to determine by further tests the accurate diagnosis of the condition; in the meantime, they issue a restrictive quarantine until the disease has been diagnosed as either an innocuous malady or one of economic importance.

The continued high level of the U.S. economy is due in part to the large numbers of healthy livestock in the nation. The *Guide for Accredited Veterinarians* (1978) quotes losses from animal diseases at approximately 1 billion dollars. Many livestock diseases of other lands do not exist here. Conversely, some nations have successfully eradicated diseases still widespread in this country, and for which no eradication programs have been authorized or undertaken to date. Veterinary Services, Animal and Plant Health Inspection Service, is alert to the shifting patterns of animal diseases. Liaisons with scientists around the world have been maintained for the development of plans to cope with emergency situations should exotic diseases find their way into the nation's livestock.

MORBIDITY AND MORTALITY REPORTING

In 1955, the USDA established a system for collecting and disseminating statistics on livestock diseases. Reporting does not, in itself, prevent the spread of disease, but it is an important foundation in building sound programs of livestock disease prevention, control, and eradication. In succeeding years, most states assumed the responsibility for collecting information within the individual states and supplying it to APHIS for the morbidity and mortality report. Statistics are collected to furnish continuing information, thereby enabling all regulatory agencies to estimate the prevalence of disease in livestock. The reports also alert regulatory officials to changes in disease incidence and provide a means to help them to plan programs for eradication of serious diseases.

Despite its laudable ambitions, however, the animal disease reporting service has several weak spots. Reports rarely show all occurrences of a given disease. To do so, all local practitioners must participate in the service, and some fail to cooperate. Further, some reports do not include all diseases observed, whereas others include some diseases more consistently than they do others. In addition, some reports may be based on incorrect field diagnoses. Additional weaknesses

are directly related to the failure of some livestock owners to consult veterinarians; thus, occurrence is not reported.

The widest possible range of accurate informational sources is needed if the final mortality and morbidity reports are to have any real meaning. Practicing veterinarians; veterinary colleges; veterinary service departments of agricultural colleges and universities; diagnostic laboratories; inspection services at public stockyards and auction markets; ante- and postmortem inspections at slaughtering plants operating under state, federal, and municipal inspection; and inspections by other regulatory officials are all important sources of useful information.

An efficient reporting system is of inestimable use in the evaluation of research requirements. It is mandatory if control and eradication programs are to receive adequate advance planning.

Modern disease-reporting techniques have many advantages. They are of material assistance in recognizing possible modes of dissemination among animal species, both wild and domestic, and they also provide indirect evidence of the effectiveness of animal disease control measures.

ANIMAL INSPECTION AND QUARANTINE

United States

The Animal Quarantine Laws are contained in the federal regulations. They are designed to prevent the spread of communicable diseases by controlling the interstate movement of livestock, including poultry, that are apparently free of diseases or exposure thereto.

The regulations also provide for the cleaning and disinfection of all cars, boats, and other vehicles used in the interstate transportation of diseased livestock and poultry. These sanitary precautions apply likewise to stockyards, holding pens, and other premises used in connection with such shipments.

Inspections for compliance with the laws are conducted throughout the United States at highway and railroad points, stockyards, and livestock centers.

Veterinary Services monitors more than 2,000 livestock concentration points for compliance with market standards and interstate regulations. Market standards for sanitation and health inspection are developed by program services staff, which administers the system of specific approval of markets complying with standards. From an economic standpoint, no service supplies more information on the health of the livestock population than does the stockyard inspection. An inspection of premises to learn which diseases exist in livestock would be an impractical and expensive procedure. A satisfactory method of making a good estimation is by inspecting animals moving through marketing centers.

This service provides a means of preventing the interstate spread of communicable diseases. It also gives buyers at inspected markets the assurance that they are getting healthy livestock.

International

International inspection and quarantine measures seek to prevent livestock diseases of foreign origin from gaining entrance into the United States as thousands of animals and millions of pounds of animal products are imported each year from all over the world.

Absolute protection against the entrance of foreign diseases through importations is impossible. The only effective measures are constant inspection and quarantine.

The United States is one of the few major livestock-producing countries of the world that remains free of devastating animal diseases prevalent in most countries.

Before necessary laws were promulgated, many animal diseases were introduced. Prior to the building of our extensive system of roads and railways, diseases did not tend to spread rapidly. However, today, with our rapid system of transport, animal diseases may quickly spread unless stringent methods of control are initiated whenever a disease of a reportable nature is discovered.

With few exceptions, animals offered for entry must be accompanied by a certificate of health issued by an official veterinarian at the point of origin. The certificate must show that the animals have been in that country for at least 60 days preceding shipment, that they have been inspected and found to be free from certain communicable diseases, and that they have not been exposed to such disease.

The responsibility for protecting the United States against foreign animal diseases has been delegated to an agency of the national government from the time of the enactment of the first legislation until today. This legislation provided for presidential authority to suspend, when necessary, any or all importations because of disease.

The Act of February 2, 1903, authorized the Secretary of Agriculture to promulgate regulations applicable to import animals and to assume other necessary measures to protect against introduction of animal disease.

Despite passage of the laws enumerated, foot-and-mouth disease gained entry into the United States nine times between 1884 and 1929. Although each epizootic was eradicated, the economic loss to the country and to the livestock producers was staggering. Without doubt, these epizootics led to legislation in 1930 that prohibited the importation of domestic ruminants and swine (and fresh, chilled, or frozen meat from all ruminants and swine) from any country declared by the Secretary of Agriculture to be infected with foot-and-mouth disease or rinderpest. In 1958, the law was amended to include a similar prohibition against wild ruminants and swine unless imported under stringent restrictions, including permanent post-entry control in USDA-approved zoologic parks.

Other statutes, previously cited, are usually referred to as the Animal Quarantine Laws. They provide the authority for imposing restrictions applicable to imported animals, animal products, hay, straw, and similar material that may transmit diseases of foreign origin, as long as such restrictions do not constitute an outright prohibition against such importations.

Because some imported animals may be carriers of latent infections, or may have been exposed to contagious or communicable diseases in transit, quarantine is maintained for a sufficiently long time to insure that the animals are free from disease or exposure. Quarantine is considered the most important step in any introduction of new animals to a herd or flock.

Control over animals intended for shipment to the United States is based primarily on a series of requirements that includes:

1. inspection and certification of the animals by a veterinarian of the national government of the country of origin.

2. knowledge about the status of animal diseases in the country of origin.

3. isolation of the animals while they are processed for shipment.

4. completion of preliminary tests as preparation for shipment.

5. a period of quarantine at the embarkation port to better insure against animals having been exposed to disease immediately prior to shipment.

6. completion of precautionary treatments if any are permitted or required.

In addition to the original health certificate issued by the veterinarian of the national government of the country of origin, a second document, a permit, provides control over the importation of animals into the United States. This is a prior permit issued by authorities in the United States to the importer. The import permit:

1. states that no other animals may be permitted aboard the transporting carrier except those for which an import permit has been issued.

2. approves the ports of call, if any, that are permitted by the carrier, and specifically forewarns that no other stops are permitted without the permit becoming invalid.

3. designates the port of arrival at which the animals must be offered for entry into the United States.

4. provides for control over the source of hay, feed, and bedding en route to eliminate possible disease exposure.

At the port of entry, Veterinary Services pass judgment on the animals being offered for entry. Control measures at the port of entry include:

1. veterinary inspection of all animals to determine that the accompanying documents are in order and that the animals appear to be free of evidence of disease or exposure thereto.

2. supervision over the cleaning and disinfection of conveyance, materials, and bedding in contact with imported animals.

3. movement of the animals from the carrier to the quarantine facilities at the port of entry, where they are supervised during their quarantine period.

4. completion of various tests required before the animals may be released from quarantine.

5. precautionary treatments that may be required while in quarantine.

6. consignment of the animals to approved destinations when appropriate.

7. supervision of disposition of animals if rejected for entry.

The restrictions on animals offered for entry into the United States are believed by some importers and others to constitute a superabundance of precautionary measures and an unnecessary duplication of effort with respect to many of the handling procedures. Nevertheless, each step is considered to be useful and necessary to insure that the United States does not become devastated by the introduction and dissemination of animal diseases of foreign origin.

The problem of disease introduction by animal products is considered by some scientists to be greater than that by the animals themselves. At present, the possibility of performing definitive diagnostic tests is greater for animals than for most animal products. Further, each animal in a shipment must be qualified with respect to tests and precautionary treatments or inspection, whereas final determination regarding imported animal products is generally, but not always, completed on a sampling basis. The import volume and complexity of both animals and products are increasing, and the advent of advanced jet-powered aircraft compounds the problems beyond any previously experienced.

CHAPTER 2

Diseases with Signs of Digestive System Changes

The diseases described in this chapter have the predominant sign of alteration of the digestive system. Other systems are affected to a degree determined by the nature and severity of the disease. Although digestive signs may be evident, there may also be concurrent signs of circulatory, respiratory, nervous, and musculoskeletal alterations. The causes of the diseases are varied and range from trauma to infection. For additional study, the following sources are suggested.

RECOMMENDED READING

Amstutz, HE: Bovine Medicine and Surgery. 2nd Edition. Chaps. 2, 3, 4, 13. Santa Barbara, CA, American Veterinary Publications, 1980.
Anderson, NV: Veterinary Gastroenterology. Philadelphia, Lea & Febiger, 1980.
Blood, DC, Henderson, JA, and Radostits, OM: Veterinary Medicine: A Textbook of the Diseases of Cattle, Sheep, Pigs, and Horses. 5th Edition. Philadelphia, Lea & Febiger, 1974.
Leman, AD, Glock, RD, Mengeling, WL, Penny, RHC, Scholl, E, and Straw, B: Diseases of Swine. 5th Edition. Chaps. 7, 13, 15, 16, 41, 42, 43, 44, 45. Ames, IA, Iowa State University Press, 1981.

Calf Scours (Neonatal Diarrhea of Calves)

Diarrhea in the early life of any animal is a dangerous condition. The term "diarrhea" is defined as a profuse watery discharge from the intestines. It is a sign of gastrointestinal disease and indicates excessive fluid loss from the body tissues. Loss of fluids and the underlying cause are difficult to control and may be fatal. There are many causes of diarrhea in newly born animals. The disease occurs more frequently wherever livestock are concentrated. Although it is a major problem for all cattle, diarrhea accounts for loss of as many as 20% of the dairy calves born.

Before a calf is born, it is sustained by the circulation of its dam. It may receive some protection against the environment from the dam before birth, but it must receive most of its protective antibodies from the colostrum of the dam after birth. Colostrum contains antibodies to the antigens to which the dam has been exposed. These antibodies protect her newborn in the same environment. Antibody levels are highest in the first milk removed from the mammary gland after calving. After removal of the first milk, antibodies progressively diminish over a period of 5 days. The newborn calf is best able to absorb the large protein molecule containing the antibody within the first 12 hours of life. Two factors then control the degree of protection a newborn calf receives; both depend on how early the calf is able to nurse and receive colostrum. It is considered that maximum benefit from colostrum is obtained by ingestion of first milk within the first hour after birth. From then on, protection diminishes in direct proportion to the time elapsed.

If the calf receives no colostrum or if the colostrum contains no protective antibodies, the calf is susceptible to the organisms in the environment. If the calf receives an overwhelming exposure to virulent organisms at the same time as it receives colostrum, the calf is still vulnerable to disease. If the calf is stressed, it is vulnerable to infection regardless of antibodies. There are specific possibilities for management of newborn calves to prevent calf scours:

1. Colostrum intake by the calf within 1 hour after birth and continued intake of colostrum for 3 to 5 days.

2. Assurance that dam is producing antibodies for protection against organisms to which the calf is exposed.

3. Control of the environment to prevent exposure to overwhelming doses of potential pathogens.

4. Prevention of stress to the calf.

Signs

The signs of calf scours may start as early as 24 hours after birth. The calf may appear normal at birth and seem strong and vigorous for several days. The first indication may be a profuse, yellow, watery diarrhea and general weakness. Appetite is diminished or absent. The muzzle becomes dry and the skin less pliable. As the diarrhea continues, the body temperature drops below normal, extremities (ears and feet) become cold, and eyes appear sunken. The skin is dry and inelastic because of loss of tissue fluid. Death may follow the onset of these signs by as few as 24 hours. The duration of the course of the disease and the onset of the first signs depend on the causative organism or circumstances.

Causes

Bacteria and viruses, individually or in combination, cause calf scours. The most common bacteria to cause calf scours is Escherichia coli. There are many strains of this organism; some are pathogenic and some are not. Some strains of E. coli are normal inhabitants of the intestines of cattle. An E. coli infection of newborn calves most often occurs in the first 3 days of life, although it can cause infection and damage later, either alone or in combination with viruses. The rotavirus and coronavirus usually cause diarrhea from the fifth to tenth day. These viruses damage the lining of the intestines and create ideal conditions for secondary bacterial infections. Salmonella bacteria affect calves as well as all species, including man. These organisms are difficult to combat and remove from the environment. Salmonella infection can occur early or late in life, even in adults. There are other organisms that can cause calf scours, but they are less frequently involved. Because so many different possible organisms can cause this disease, it is understandable how signs, time of occurrence, and degree of severity can be so varied.

Transmission

The route of infection for organisms causing calf scours is through the mouth of the calf. It can also enter the umbilicus of the newborn. If the calf is born in an environment that is contaminated by potential infectious bacteria, the likelihood of its contracting the disease is increased. The repeated use of the same area, barn lot, small pasture, or stall for delivering calves frequently results in contamination by feces. Cattle feces contain E. coli or other potential pathogens. In pastures, cows have a tendency to seclude themselves in lower, poorly drained areas for calving. Sometimes sheltered areas become badly contaminated. Often, to facilitate close observation, a small pasture close to the farmhouse is used continuously for calving. Or, in spite of the good intention to have ideal maternity stalls in a barn, these stalls are frequently not kept clean and become a source of infection. So, the calf's introduction into the world is accompanied by a bath of organisms that can cause a fatal disease. When the newborn first nurses to receive protective colostrum, the udder and teats of the cow could be badly contaminated from lying in filth. The calf then receives a dose of pathogens too great to be overcome by the colostrum it is consuming.

Of course, a calf can become infected even when calving areas are controlled. The dairy calf removed from the dam is frequently placed in an environment that is already contaminated by previous calves or is placed in contact with calves already infected. Or, the utensils, calf bucket, or nipple bottle used to feed the calves are contaminated. The milk or milk replacer can also be contaminated.

Prevention and Control

Prevention and control of calf scours depend on the four management possibilities mentioned previously.

1. Intake of colostrum to transfer antibodies from the dam to the calf must be assured. Even though constant surveillance of cows during calving may not seem practical, colostrum must be received early to give the calf the best chance for survival. Finding a newborn the "morning after" and helping it to nurse is not as effective as either helping it to nurse the first hour or milking the colostrum from the cow and force-feeding it to the calf. The use of a calf

feeder with an esophageal tube attached to a plastic bag is becoming a common practice. Leaving the calf with the cow and assuming that it will get colostrum is risky. The effort required to be certain of colostrum intake must be evaluated in relation to the value of the calf. Because early intake of colostrum is so important for survival of calves, some calf buyers insist that a simple blood test be performed to indicate colostrum intake. Decisions to buy are made on the basis of the test results.

2. To assure that colostrum has all the antibodies necessary for survival of the calf, one must consider several factors. One can assume that, if the cow has been in her current environment for most of her life, she will have antibodies to most of the potential pathogens. However, a recently acquired cow from another environment may not have the antibodies to the organisms that will challenge her calf in the new environment. It is also possible that the cow will not have antibodies to some of the viruses that affect calves. Therefore, cows must be vaccinated with these virus vaccines in advance of calving to attempt to build immunity and possible colostrum antibodies. These same vaccines can be given to the calf at birth in an attempt to block infection by the viruses.

An additional problem arises for the calf that is removed from its dam and placed in an environment never experienced by the cow. Even if this calf has antibodies from its dam, it may not be protected against organisms in a calf barn or facility where calves from several sources are collected. The calf protected by colostrum still needs the additional protection of strict sanitation in such a facility.

3. Control of the environment during and after calving requires no additional discussion except to emphasize that newborn calves cannot survive the overwhelming challenge of excessive contamination. Investigators have conclusively proved the value of clean, dry, maternity stalls in the prevention of calf scours. Although the navel of a calf should be dipped and soaked in 7% tincture of iodine immediately after birth, even this cannot combat a bath in filth and feces.

4. The final management possibility is prevention of stress. Calves can be stressed and weakened by exposure to cold, rain, snow, excessive heat, or humidity. They can also be stressed by overfeeding or underfeeding. The wet, chilled calf is more susceptible to scours. The overfed calf may develop nutritional scours, which predispose the calf to infection. Control over the elements has practical limitations. Clean, dry, individual hutches are considered ideal for dairy calves. The use of slatted floors or a series of wire cages facilitates feeding and waste removal but can be hazardous because of dampness or exposure to draft.

Calves can nurse too much. High-producing beef cows on lush pasture could cause a nutritional scouring in calves. More often, however, the dairy calf is overfed. Recommended colostrum intake is 4 pounds in the first 12 hours. Thereafter, the milk or colostrum intake should be approximately 5% of the body weight per day, gradually reaching a maximum of about 1 gallon per day until weaning. When milk replacers are used, the manufacturer's recommendations should be followed closely.

Treatment

Treatment for neonatal diarrhea in the calf has undergone dramatic changes during the past 10 years. Instead of being directed toward stopping the diarrhea with drugs that slow down gut activity and coat the inflamed lining, treatment has become directed toward replacement of the fluid and electrolyte loss. Counteracting the lethal effects of dehydration has sustained the sick calf long enough to recover from the disease. By the use of a balanced electrolyte solution containing dextrose, given orally instead of milk, the tissues can be rehydrated. The electrolyte solution can be given for as many as 5 days as a substitute for milk or milk replacer. Concurrent treatment with antibiotics directed toward the specific organism may be necessary. Selec-

tion of the antibiotic should be based on results from laboratory cultures. In some cases, it may be possible to diagnose the cause accurately from the type of diarrhea and other signs.

Digestive System Diseases of Swine

Swine production is adversely affected by many diseases of the digestive system. Although the cause of some of these diseases may be primarily diet, an infectious agent is involved in most. As expected, diseases affecting baby pigs are severe and result in high mortality. Prominent digestive system diseases of swine are colibacillosis, edema disease, transmissible gastroenteritis, salmonellosis, and swine dysentery. All these are of economic significance and need to be controlled. There has been and continues to be extensive research for effective means of control. Although the following discussion of some of these diseases is brief and in summary form, the reader is cautioned to realize that there are no simple answers to the control problems involved.

COLIBACILLOSIS

Colibacillosis is an acute disease of baby pigs that affects the stomach and intestines, causing a yellow, watery diarrhea. Mortality is high from the toxemia and septicemia that result. The disease spreads rapidly within a litter and is transmitted within a farrowing house by contact with anything contaminated by the feces of infected pigs.

Signs

There are several possibilities. The pigs may become sick and die within 48 hours after birth with no signs of a diarrhea. They sometimes are noticed first to be

weak, dull, and dehydrated after developing a diarrhea; they then die. If the pigs get some immunity from colostrum, they may not show signs until several weeks after birth, when a diarrhea develops.

Cause

The cause is exposure to a pathogenic serotype of Escherichia coli. This organism is a normal inhabitant of the digestive tract of all species. If it occurs in sufficient numbers and is of a virulent type to which there is no resistance, the pigs may absorb the toxins and the organisms, thereby developing a septicemia and toxemia. Because feces carry E. coli, this organism is present and available to the mouth of the newborn from the sow's udder, the floor, bedding, and utensils.

Diagnosis

Colibacillosis must be differentiated from other neonatal diarrhea diseases, such as transmissible gastroenteritis (TGE). Sometimes the history of its occurrence is valuable. TGE occurs most often in cold months, whereas colibacillosis is not seasonal. TGE is characterized by vomiting and colibacillosis is not. Necropsy and histopathologic signs differ. TGE can be diagnosed by use of a fluorescent antibody test. The morbidity and mortality of TGE in pigs under 1 week of age is close to 100%. This is not so with colibacillosis, which may be limited to certain litters, or to only some pigs in a litter. Sows may show mild signs of TGE.

Prevention and Control

There are two avenues of approach to the prevention of colibacillosis. The first is to reduce the number of organisms available for exposure. The second is to increase the resistance of the pigs to the organism.

The number of organisms available for exposure can be reduced by rigid sanitation in the farrowing house, washing the sow's udder before farrowing, steam cleaning of the farrowing house between farrowings, and strict control over visitors. Sanitation as a preventive measure by itself requires careful and intense management. Sanitation should be combined with elimination of stress factors, such as damp floors, excessive humidity, and drafts. Further reduction of exposure can be accomplished by maintaining a closed herd or, if swine are added, by isolating them from the herd for at least 30 days.

Increased resistance to infection can be accomplished by immunization. Because of the variety of serotypes of E. coli that may cause infection, immunization by commercially prepared vaccines has not been completely effective. Practices to provide the sow with prior exposure to the types of organisms in the farrowing environment to be used are effective. Exposing the sow and allowing time (3 to 4 weeks) for development of antibodies provides protection to her pigs via colostrum. This has been done in several ways:

1. By allowing free contact by sows and gilts with the farrowing facilities and each other before and after breeding.

2. By putting bred sows in the farrowing house at least 3 weeks before farrowing.

3. By exposing sows to the farrowing facilities by periodic 1- or 2-day visits to the farrowing house 3 or more weeks before farrowing.

4. By collecting feces from pigs with a diarrhea in the farrowing pens, and mixing with sow feed 30 days before farrowing.

These practices risk transmitting to the sow viruses that cause other diseases. It is also advisable to contaminate sow feed with feces of pigs under 8 weeks of age to avoid ingestion of parasite eggs. A better practice is the use of specifically prepared autogenous vaccines from the strains of the organism in the farrowing house. These vaccines can be added to the sow's feed 3 weeks before farrowing.

Treatment

Treatment is never satisfactory because of the rapid dehydration and weakness from diarrhea. However, a variety of antibiotics have been and are being used to reduce the infection in the baby pigs. Oral administration of antibiotics is considered more effective than injection. Oral dosing or adding of sulfonamides or furacin to the pigs' drinking water has been successful at times. Altering the flora for the infecting organism by adding Lactobacillus acidophilus to milk and feeding it to the pigs has been effective in preventing or reducing the severity of diarrhea.

Because response to therapy is so variable and the effort is so time consuming, means of prevention by immunization and sanitation are of primary concern.

EDEMA DISEASE

Edema disease, or gut edema, is an acute disease of young swine characterized by sudden onset, incoordination, and swelling of various tissues of the body.

The most susceptible period is weaning time or shortly thereafter and appears to be related to such stress factors as the radical change in feeding at this time, castration, and vaccination against other diseases. The most typical manifestation, and the most useful diagnostically, is a staggering gait, which is considered to be a toxic manifestation.

Although edema disease in pigs was first described in North Ireland in 1938, its wide distribution and economic importance have been recognized only recently. Currently, the disease has been diagnosed in the United States, Canada, South Africa, and most countries in Europe, and there is reason to believe that it exists in many other countries where it is either undiagnosed or confused with some other condition.

Edema disease typically affects pigs 8 to 16 weeks of age and within 7 to 10 days after weaning. The disease frequently follows a change of diet. It has been observed following vaccination for hog cholera.

Cause

The attention of several investigators has been directed to the disease because of its economic importance and its considerable academic interest. Efforts have been made to determine the specific cause of the disease so that it might be controlled by prophylactic means. The cause has remained obscure for a long time, and numerous possibilities have been suggested. One theory is that the disease may be a specific toxemia originating either in the digestive tract or from the ingestion of a preformed toxin. The signs and lesions of edema disease have been produced experimentally by the supernatant fluid from centrifuged intestinal contents of affected animals and by saline extracts of the same material. This observation provides evidence that a specific enterotoxemia originating in the intestines can cause the disease.

Because of the predominance of hemolytic Escherichia coli in the intestinal contents of affected animals, a relationship between this organism and the disease has been postulated. The rapidly growing E. coli organisms invade the intestinal epithelium, and their endotoxins are absorbed into the systemic circulation. The endotoxins could therefore exert a damaging influence on the nervous and vascular systems and, thereby, produce characteristic signs and lesions of the disease. There is also some evidence to support the idea that anaphylaxis is the cause.

Signs

Onset of the disease is sudden, with a mortality of 50 to 70%. Sometimes the course is rapid, and pigs may die without showing previous signs of illness. Affected pigs may or may not have an increase in body temperature. Diarrhea is not a consistent sign. Some pigs may be constipated.

Edema in various sites is a characteristic finding useful to diagnosis. Edema of the eyelids, the ears, and the face occurs commonly. Pigs appear to lose muscular control; they display a staggering gait and knuckling of the forelegs. When a pig becomes recumbent, it usually exhibits running movements and muscular twitching. The grunt or squeal is abnormal. Some pigs, if left undisturbed and quiet, recover in 24 to 48 hours. Others continue the nervous signs until death occurs. Affected pigs kept with the rest of the herd are usually abused by the healthy pigs and will die unless removed to a protected, quiet area.

When a postmortem examination is made soon after death, a remarkable amount of edematous fluid frequently is found in the gastric or intestinal submucosa and the colonic mesentery. The stomach, which usually is full of food, has a wall thickened from the accumulation of edematous exudate. The lymph nodes may be grossly swollen from congestion and edema. The gallbladder, perirenal areas, lungs, subcutaneous tissues, and nervous system also may be markedly edematous.

Diagnosis

Diagnosis is based on the history, clinical signs, and necropsy findings. The only pathogen that may be found is E. coli. The absence of signs of other diseases is helpful in the final diagnosis.

Prevention

No suitable prophylactic bacterin or vaccine is available. Radical changes in diet and other stresses routinely imposed on growing pigs at weaning should be eliminated when possible. Feeding changes can lead to fatal consequences. A transitional diet at weaning can establish a new balance without causing rapid changes in intestinal flora which might encourage the development of the microorganisms suspected in this disease.

Treatment

There is no satisfactory treatment. Saline laxatives and a reduced diet seem to be helpful. Drugs administered to combat the toxemia, such as corticosteroids and antihistamines, have been tried with little success.

TRANSMISSIBLE GASTROENTERITIS (TGE)

Transmissible gastroenteritis (TGE) of swine is an extremely contagious and fatal viral disease. All ages of swine are affected. Pigs under 2 weeks of age have almost 100% mortality, whereas those 5 weeks of age and older usually survive. Mature sows and boars are affected, but rarely have more than a mild diarrhea of a few days' duration.

TGE is a disease exclusive to swine. The virus is not known to affect other species of animals. Although first recognized in the United States, it is now reported to occur in much of Europe, Canada, Japan, and Taiwan. Because of the high mortality in baby pigs and the rapid spread, the disease is of considerable economic importance to the swine industry.

Signs

Vomiting and diarrhea are consistent and characteristic in pigs under 2 weeks of age. Pigs may vomit, nurse, and then vomit again. The diarrhea is yellow and watery and may contain particles of undigested milk. The course and duration are rapid for pigs several days old. Weakness, dehydration, and death may take place within 24 hours. In general, pigs under 10 days of age usually die within 2 to 7 days after initial signs. Some veterinarians have

observed a variation in the severity of the disease from year to year. Such a variation could be attributed to changes in the virulence of the virus. However, because of the similarity of its signs to those of colibacillosis or other causes of diarrhea, the diagnosis may be inaccurate.

Signs for older pigs, sows, and boars become increasingly mild as the animal ages. Sows may have a slight rise in body temperature, lose their appetite for 24 hours, and have a diarrhea for several days. It is possible, but not likely, that sows nursing pigs will become agalactic from the disease.

Cause

TGE is caused by a virus that affects the lining of the stomach and intestines. Damage to the intestinal epithelium is so severe that absorption of nutrients and electrolytes is prevented. The virus is eliminated with feces and invades other pigs either orally or by inhalation. The virus is stable in the frozen state and fairly labile at 70° F or higher. When frozen, it can be maintained viable for 18 months.

Diagnosis

Vomiting, diarrhea, and death in very young pigs are characteristic diagnostic signs. These signs, coupled with the explosive spread to other pigs and high mortality in those under 2 weeks of age, are strong indications of TGE. Necropsy of affected pigs usually discloses markedly distended blood vessels in the mesentery and hyperemia of the lining of the small intestines. Characteristic cell changes can be observed by microscopic examination. Other laboratory tests to determine the presence of the virus can be used for a definite diagnosis.

Control and Prevention

Active immunity resulting from natural infection or by vaccination with the live virus has been disappointing. However, pigs nursing recovered sows receive sufficient passive immunity from colostrum to withstand challenge by live virus for almost a year. Therefore, the best protection for the baby pig is to nurse a mother that has been infected and has recovered 2 to 3 weeks prior to farrowing.

Because the virus survives best in cold weather, most severe outbreaks occur during the winter when the virus can be transported by any object carrying infected feces from one group of pigs to another. Birds, shoes or boots of workers, and barn cleaning equipment have been known to transport the virus. Strict control of farrowing-unit sanitation is necessary, as is control of visitors. Feces from recovered swine carry the virus for several months in progressively lesser quantities.

If threatened with an outbreak, a recommended plan for control is:

1. Feed infected material to sows 3 to 4 weeks before farrowing.

2. If sows are within 2 weeks of farrowing when the outbreak occurs, move them to isolation in unexposed facilities and, if possible, prevent any contact by the personnel working with the infected unit.

Immunization by vaccines is considered to have some value in developing antibodies in sows if administered well in advance of farrowing.

Treatment

All manner of therapy to restore fluid and electrolyte balance to pigs under 2 weeks of age has been of little value in preventing losses. The use of oral antibiotics to prevent secondary bacterial infections may be of some value in older pigs.

Salmonellosis

Salmonellosis is an acute or chronic contagious disease caused by one or more species of bacteria of the genus Salmonella. Salmonellosis is characterized by moderate fever, profuse hemorrhagic diarrhea, gastroenteritis, respiratory difficulties, intense septicemia, and, in some cases, a prolonged state of unthriftiness. Salmonellae have been isolated from outbreaks of infection in all the common domestic animals and man. Several hundred species of Salmonella are capable of producing infection in mammals, birds, fish, reptiles, and, particularly, rodents. Among the various strains, certain species tend to be host adaptive, whereas others show no host adaptation at all.

Geographically, salmonellosis is worldwide in distribution and is found particularly where swine and cattle are maintained in crowded conditions. Within the United States, salmonellosis is more common in the corn belt of the middle west than in other parts of the country. However, the disease is universal in distribution and is found wherever animals are found.

Historically, salmonellosis is one of the oldest reported diseases of swine. The true nature of the condition was not discovered until 1885, when it was described as being identified with hog cholera. However, with the isolation of the viral cause of hog cholera in the early 1900s, the true nature of the disease associated with Salmonella organisms was discovered. Salmonellosis in cattle was first observed in the United States in 1902, and has since been found in all parts of the country and in other countries where cattle are maintained.

Cause

Salmonellosis in livestock can be caused by one or more species of Salmonella. The most prevalent cause in cattle is Salmonella typhimurium, closely followed by S. dublin and S. newport. The most prevalent cause of the disease in swine is S. choleraesuis. Although the pig is considered the reservoir for S. choleraesuis, this species has also been recovered from man, cattle, dogs, poultry, and wild animals. The disease is more common in young animals than in adult animals. The mortality is much higher in the young than in the old, although both young and adult animals may frequently be debilitated. Carrier animals exist among adults, and the infection may persist in an inapparent form in these animals for many years. Such animals, however, may develop active clinical signs if subjected to stressful conditions, such as inclement weather, poor nutrition, and other infectious diseases causing debilitation.

Transmission

The primary route of infection for salmonellosis is through the alimentary tract. The infective bacteria are introduced into the alimentary tract through contaminated feed and water. Animals actively excreting the microorganisms during the acute stage of the disease, or carrier animals excreting the microorganisms, are primary sources of infection. Secondarily, feed contaminated by urine and fecal material of rodents is a frequent source of spread of salmonellosis.

This disease may be considered to be associated with mismanagement in relation to its transmission to young animals. Young calves and pigs maintained in less-than-optimum sanitary conditions, associated with older animals, and crowded into filthy barnyards or holding yards are particularly susceptible to the disease through the bacteria deposited in the soil by fecal material of older carrier animals.

There is little evidence that prenatal infection occurs with this disease. However, if the dam is suffering from clinical salmonellosis during parturition (indicated by acute diarrhea, high temperature, low milk yield, and almost complete loss of appetite), she is likely to be excreting salmonellae in the colostrum. The number of animals affected in this manner is low; observations of clinically normal dams soon after parturition show salmonellae in the feces, on the udder, and on the teat surfaces, but not in the milk. In most instances, young animals obtain the infective microorganisms from the surface of the teats while nursing. Salmonellae may often be demonstrated in the feces within 24 to 36 hours after birth.

In addition to direct dam-to-offspring transmission, Salmonella microorganisms in the environment of young animals can result in infant infection at an early age. Usually, recently born calves and piglets are brought into a shed, barnyard, or holding area for preliminary inspection. Calves are often placed in small enclosures for varying periods of time. After a day or two, the cow may return to the herd. The calf is allowed to suckle only for a short period before being sent to slaughter or mixed with older calves. Young pigs, however, are usually confined in a farrowing area in a barn or shed that has been used for many previous farrowings and may not be as sanitary as it should be. These maternity and/or feeding areas usually get perennially heavy traffic, and if adults in the herd are excreting Salmonella, the enclosures can quickly become grossly contaminated. Furthermore, these areas usually favor persistence of the microorganisms. Observations on premises where outbreaks have occurred show that, in most instances, the feeding equipment is grossly contaminated, as are the water troughs and containers.

Without equivocation, however, the most persistent means by which salmonellosis is transmitted is the carrier animal. Carriers seed the soil and equipment within an area with the microorganisms for direct and indirect transmission to susceptible animals. The bacteria causing salmonellosis in livestock may also cause food poisoning in humans from foodstuffs containing the organisms from fecal-contaminated hands.

Factors Influencing Susceptibility

Observation for the presence of Salmonella microorganisms were made on both calves and pigs sent to slaughterhouses. In most instances, the mixing and mingling of hogs held in the pens at sale barns and in holding pens at packing plants provided the means for extensive exposure and spread of salmonella from animal to animal; salmonellae were isolated from the drinking water of the pens and from the feed containers. At slaughter, animals were found to be contaminated by Salmonella species highly pathogenic to man.

Overcrowding of young calves, particularly during inclement weather in poor housing, is also conducive to the spread of infection. Some calf enclosures are unsatisfactory because regular or even inefficient cleaning is virtually impossible. When housing cannot be readily cleaned, particularly between groups of calves, it is advisable to resort to some sort of temporary shelter.

Excessive crowding during transportation is another means by which salmonellosis is readily transmitted. There is no evidence that debilitated animals are more likely than apparently healthy animals to harbor salmonellae; therefore, animals maintained in overcrowded, unsanitary conditions probably are exposed to excessively high numbers of Salmonella microorganisms and transmit them with regularity.

Recent evidence shows that young calves can excrete more organisms than can older calves. Consequently, the importance of initially isolating young or recently bought calves from older animals is evident. The isolated calves are likely to obtain better supervision, particularly when being taught to drink or when requiring treatment. Young calves should be fed with separate utensils, and isolation pens or sheds should be cleaned and disinfected between groups of animals. Purchase of calves in small groups directly from another property minimizes the risk of acquiring infective animals.

Salmonellosis may develop in feedlot cattle any time in the fattening period, but it occurs also in adult dairy cows and, still more frequently, in calves. While the disease may occur during any month of the year, its incidence is highest from June through October. Age is a definite factor influencing susceptibility to salmonellosis; however, breed and sex are not significant. Salmonellosis is more prevalent in dairy animals than in beef cattle, primarily because of manner of management. In the western range herds in particular, salmonellosis is seldom seen until animals are segregated by age groups for transport to market.

Clinical Signs

Salmonella infections in all species of mammals are characterized by fever, recumbency, and gastrointestinal upsets. The clinical infection may be acute or chronic.

Acute salmonellosis in swine affects primarily young animals from 3 weeks to 6 months of age. The most common signs of infection are obvious debility and depression, refusal to eat, and an increase in temperature to 104 to 106° F with a rapid rate of respiration. Some animals may not demonstrate diarrhea, although this is usually a predominant feature of the disease. In field cases, the animal shows a rough, staring hair coat, a rapid loss of weight, and dehydration caused by persistent diarrhea. Some animals die in 2 to 4 days; others may survive and either recover or pass into the chronic phase, during which their continued growth rate is relatively slow.

In the chronic phase in swine, survivors of the acute type develop slowly. They may have a persistent diarrhea, which is yellow in color, semiliquid in consistency, and has an offensive odor. They have moderate fever and may stand with tucked-up abdomen and eat sparsely. When forced to move, the animals groan, grunt, and squeal with reluctance. They may either lose weight rapidly or gain poorly. Some have persistent respiratory distress and may not live longer than several weeks, although others consistently shed the bacteria until they reach advanced age in rather poor, thin condition.

Acute salmonellosis in calves occurs suddenly, with a temperature of 105 to 108° F. Diarrhea is evident on the second day of infection. Dehydration, weakness, and loss of appetite appear in most affected calves by the third day. In the severe acute cases, the feces frequently are watery in consistency, yellowish in color, and fetid in odor. The calves show depression, dehydration, and rapid loss of weight; death occurs in 3 to 7 days, depending on the severity of the symptoms.

In a milking herd, the disease progresses rapidly with a drastic drop in milk production, severe diarrhea, dehydration, and extreme lassitude. Temperatures are usually elevated above 105° F but seldom persist for more than 2 days before dropping to a lower level, although still higher than normal. Pregnant cows may abort, and death may occur in 2 to 4 days depending on the severity of the symptoms.

In the chronic phase, the clinical form is usually seen in calves in which pneumonia and arthritis may complicate the picture. Sporadic outbreaks are seen only in older cattle. Subclinical salmonellosis may occur in bovines of all ages, however. Adult animals recovering from the acute clinical disease tend to excrete the organisms in their feces for a considerable length of time. S. dublin infections tend to persist for particularly long periods, S. typhimurium persist for shorter periods, and other species last for only a few days. Calves usually do not remain carriers after recovery. Salmonellae are excreted in the milk of lactating cows only in the febrile stage of the disease.

In general, the signs observed in an outbreak of salmonellosis in any mammals resemble those of acute septicemic disease. Milder forms of the infection accompanied by indefinite signs do occur, and it is quite possible that some animals become carriers of the disease without showing any visible signs.

Postmortem Signs

After ingestion, the microorganisms rapidly invade the body; they have been found on slaughter in the lungs, lymph nodes, and blood of infected animals. In the intestine, bacteria proliferate and cause severe injury to the mucosa. Necrosis of epithelial cells and erosion of blood vessels cause hemorrhaging into the intestinal lumen. Irritation to the intestine provokes diarrhea early in the course of the disease. Some bacteria may penetrate the blood vessels to produce septicemia and foci of infection in the liver, spleen, and lymph nodes. After a short course, death may result from dehydration, hemorrhaging, intoxication, and septicemia. Postmortem lesions in swine usually include bright red mucosa of the stomach, covered with a thin film of tenacious mucus. Some necrosis is always present. The most consistent postmortem lesion is a severe gastroenteritis. The spleen is enlarged, dark blue, and firm and swollen. Hemorrhages may appear in the renal cortex, on the heart, and on the mucous membranes of the intestinal tract. The contents of the intestinal tract are fluid and may contain blood. In cases of severe intestinal hemorrhaging, anemia is present. All animal tissues may be dehydrated.

Diagnosis

In the field, the diagnosis of salmonellosis is based primarily on herd history, prior vaccination status, and clinical signs. Profuse diarrhea with blood in the feces is highly significant. In cattle, one of the premonitory signs is failure to respond to treatment for other conditions resembling this disease. A laboratory confirmation may be obtained by isolation and identification of salmonellae from fecal samples and from lymph nodes of animals that have died in the herd or flock. If an animal or aborted fetus is infected with Salmonella, the organisms are easy to isolate.

Prevention

Preventive measures are important. The primary consideration in preventing salmonellosis is adequate sanitation. Livestock should be maintained in clean lots, and pastures should be rotated to prevent a buildup of fecal material containing pathogenic bacteria. The introduction of infected animals into a herd or flock should be avoided at all costs. Calves should be segregated by age group during the growing period because the most common manner of spreading the disease is mixing young animals with older animals that are inapparent spreaders of the bacteria.

Other diseases causing primary infection and lowering resistance should be prevented when possible.

Modern methods of sanitation, proper nutrition, and good management should be exercised. Such practices allow the operator to maintain the health and vigor of his animals. When proper immunization methods are available, animals should be vaccinated on a routine basis.

In an effort to control the contamination of indigenous foodstuffs that may have a bearing on transmission of salmonellosis, either to livestock or to human beings, U.S. Department of Agriculture in cooperation with the various states has initiated an eradication and testing program. The program has been published in a set of regulations entitled, "Uniform Methods and Rules for the Elimination of Salmonella in Animal By-Products Intended for Use in Animal Feeds." It is recommended by the U.S. Animal Health Association, and became effective January 8, 1969. A copy of the regulations may be obtained from state or federal regulatory veterinarians or agricultural extension agents.

Several commercially available bacterins may be used to protect livestock against a specific species of Salmonella. However, most bacterins are of questionable efficiency, and care should be taken not to rely entirely on such prophylaxis. Mixed bacterins are available that confer a degree of resistance against infection by the organisms represented in the formula. The degree of resistance, however, is enhanced by a series of injections at 2- to 3-week intervals; usually, about 3 injections are required. Increased sensitivity to antigens may be a problem with repeated injections, and care should be taken to prevent anaphylactic shock or to treat it if it occurs.

Treatment

Sick animals require help early in the course of the disease if they are to survive. Antibiotics administered either by injection to individual animals or in water or feed to large groups are effective.

Bovine Virus Diarrhea

Bovine virus diarrhea is an acute or chronic contagious and infectious disease of cattle characterized by fever, nasal discharge, coughing, profuse watery diarrhea, rapid dehydration, and emaciation.

Bovine virus diarrhea was first described in New York in 1946 and has been found since that time by serological survey to be widespread through all countries where cattle are produced. Up to 56% of adult cattle have antibodies to this virus, and it is difficult to find baby calves, either dairy or beef, without demonstrable antibodies.

Cause

Bovine virus diarrhea is caused by one of several strains of a virus. All strains are serologically and immunologically related, although some are cytopathogenic whereas others are not. Manifestations of the disease vary for each strain of the virus. The causative agent propagates in cell cultures of sheep, goats, cattle, and embryonating egg.

Bovine virus diarrhea occurs at all times of the year. It principally affects young cattle, from 8 months to 2 years of age, of both dairy and beef breeds; however, it has also been observed in aged cattle. A few cases on record indicate, by clinical manifestations and by the demonstration of ascending bovine virus diarrhea antibody titers on paired serum samples, that the disease can occur in baby calves 1 to 4 weeks of age. A strong antigenic relationship exists between this virus and the virus of hog cholera.

Transmission

The mode of transmission is thought to be direct contact from infected to susceptible cattle, but the exact method of transfer is not known. The virus may be transmitted indirectly by contaminated feed, water, and bedding, and by contact with fecal matter during the stage of viremia. The disease often appears in a herd after the addition of replacement cattle or after subjection to the stress of shipment. Subacute signs appear in 1 or 2 animals, followed in a week to 10 days by a fulminating outbreak in the herd.

Clinical Signs

Bovine virus diarrhea is characterized by a chain of signs initially of a respiratory nature: serous or mucous nasal discharge, labored breathing, coughing, and elevated temperatures. In addition, an affected animal usually appears gaunt as a result of decreased feed consumption and diarrhea. Acute laminitis occurs occasionally. Other signs include fatal anomalies, weak calves, muscular tremors, and incoordination. Bovine virus diarrhea has a course of several days in adult dairy cattle. The course in feedlot cattle, on an individual basis, is usually from 10 days to 2 or 3 weeks in acute outbreaks and from 4 to 6 weeks on a lot basis. Chronic cases extend over a period of months, and affected cattle are finally sold or eventually die.

Although the morbidity is generally high, the mortality is low. The loss is primarily economic because of weight loss, prolonged feeding periods, chronic sickness, abortions, loss of milk production, proprietary drug costs, and fees for veterinary diagnostic laboratory services.

The onset often is sudden, with temperatures ranging from 104 to 106° F. Because cattle can appear well with a high fever, the temperatures of several animals in the herd should be checked. Depression is moderate to severe; respirations and pulse are rapid. Affected cattle have almost no appetite; however, they drink large amounts of water.

Moderate to severe nasal discharge occurs shortly after onset and may be accompanied by a low, throaty, unproductive cough. The nasal discharge is serous at first but, in chronic cases, may become mucopurulent and, in severe cases, can cover the entire muzzle. The nasal mucosa may show marked hyperemia, and at this stage, the disease may be confused with infectious bovine rhinotracheitis or even shipping fever. In some outbreaks, there may be many subclinical cases.

Excessive lacrimation is sometimes seen and may be followed by a progressive corneal opacity. In some cases, oral lesions are found early in the course of the disease. They usually are uneven, round or shallow erosions, but may consist only of areas of congestion. They are most common on the dental pad, inner surface of the lips, and buccal mucosa. Similar lesions are sometimes found on the muzzle and in the nares.

Lameness, apparently caused by laminitis, is seen in the severe cases and is characterized by a peculiar stance. The soreness causes many cattle to lie down more frequently than usual. In severe cases, the tissues around the coronary band of the feet are severely reddened.

During the early febrile stage, the feces are hard and dry, and may be covered with mucus and a few flecks of blood. Diarrhea may occur in about 10% of cases.

When present, it begins after the peak of the febrile response has passed and may continue intermittently for 4 to 6 weeks or even longer. The feces are watery and fetid, containing many bubbles and long strings of mucus; they vary from yellowish to slate gray to red, when more erythrocytes are present. Because diarrhea occurs so inconsistently in affected cattle, the term "virus diarrhea" may be considered somewhat of a misnomer.

Dehydration is severe, and some affected animals lose considerable body weight. The eyes are dull and sunken, and the skin becomes dry and scurfy. The skin changes are particularly severe on the neck.

A few younger animals may have convulsions prior to death. Death is most likely to occur early in the course of the disease. In severely affected cattle that recover, convalescence is protracted and often causes as much or more economic loss as does death. The course of the disease is milder in small calves and in older animals. In these animals mild respiratory involvement and diarrhea may lead to unthriftiness, and temperatures may not rise above 102 to 103.5° F.

There are three distinct forms of bovine virus diarrhea. The *inapparent* form is evidenced by mild symptoms and slightly elevated temperature. However, because of the diphasic temperature pattern, the clinical examination may reveal a temperature of from 102 to 107° F without serious complications.

The *acute or severe* form is sudden in onset and involves an entire herd with the full gamut of symptoms.

The *chronic* form is likely to be an extension of the inapparent form. It is characterized by rough hair coat, poor condition, persistent nasal discharge, failure to gain weight, and lameness.

Postmortem Signs

Lesions occur primarily in the alimentary tract and adjacent lymphatic tissues; they are hemorrhages, inflammation, edema, and shallow irregular erosions of the mucosal lining. Oral lesions occur in only a small percentage of diseased cattle. Ulcerative lesions are extensive throughout the gastrointestinal tract and in the buccal cavity. Inflammation, edema, hemorrhages, and ulcers, in various stages of formation and repair, are found consistently in the abomasum. Occasionally, there are erosions on the pillars of the rumen. Usually there is a catarrhal enteritis with some erosions of the lining, and subserous edema often occurs around the small intestine. The lymph glands adjacent to the gastrointestinal tract may be enlarged and edematous.

Diagnosis

A presumptive diagnosis can be made from clinical evidence and postmortem lesions. A definitive diagnosis can be made by isolating the virus from nasal discharges and blood during the acute febrile phase, before circulating antibodies are formed. The virus can also be isolated from the spleen and mesenteric lymph glands.

The most practical way to arrive at a definitive diagnosis is serologic. Cross-protection or serum neutralization studies can be made with paired-serum samples. The first or acute blood samples should be taken when the sick animal is first observed. A second or convalescent blood sample should be taken 2 to 3 weeks later and processed the same way. Ideally, there will be no bovine virus diarrhea antibodies in the first serum sample, whereas the second will contain demonstrable antibodies.

It is not unusual for cattle vaccinated against infectious bovine rhinotracheitis to undergo an attack of bovine virus diarrhea. This causes the owner and/or the veterinarian to think they are experiencing an infectious bovine rhinotracheitis immunity failure. At times, both diseases have been found to be active not only in the same lot of cattle but in the same animal.

The disease most difficult to differentiate and most often confused with bovine virus diarrhea (BVD) is infectious bovine rhinotracheitis (IBR). Clinically, IBR is a respiratory disease in feedlot cattle, whereas BVD is an enteric disease. Laminitis, frequently seen in BVD, is not a part of IBR. The suppurative, palpebral conjunctivitis of IBR does not involve the eyeball, whereas that of BVD occasionally does. Corneal opacity with keratitis, seen in BVD, is not seen in IBR conjunctivitis on a lot basis.

Prevention

The virus of BVD is ubiquitous. As a result, 60 to 80% of all cattle have antibodies to the virus. Those that do not have antibodies are either incapable of developing antibodies or have never been exposed to the virus. Because the disease is so widespread and can cause economic losses through abortions, weak or deformed calves, unthrifty cattle, and death loss, protection provided by vaccination is usually necessary. The exception to vaccination would be in the closed herd in which the disease has never been diagnosed and whose area is free of the disease.

Current recommendations are to vaccinate calves 6 to 8 months of age with any of the commercial vaccines available. Results of vaccination have raised questions as to the efficacy and safety of the vaccines. Questions raised include possible vaccine causes of abortion if used on pregnant animals, the effect of vaccines during a herd outbreak, and apparent lack of protection by the vaccine. Colostral antibodies in calves under 6 months of age interfere with development of active immunity. Also, some cattle do not develop antibodies from either natural exposure or vaccines.

To avoid the possibility of causing abortion by vaccination, some recommend that heifers be vaccinated at least 30 days prior to breeding. And, if annual revaccination is necessary, it should be done to open cows at least 30 days prior to rebreeding.

Because vaccines are constantly being changed and improved, many of the questions currently raised will be invalid in the future.

Treatment

There is no specific treatment for cattle affected by BVD. Appropriate supportive therapy to nourish and rehydrate severely sick animals and antibiotics to suppress secondary bacterial infection are indicated. Treatment of the acute and chronically affected cattle is disappointing. Treatment of mild or subclinical disease is unnecessary.

Bloat

Bloat, or tympanites, is a specific disease of ruminants that causes an annual loss to producers of millions of dollars. It is characterized by retention of gas in the rumen, with consequent overextension of the abdomen from pressures produced within the rumen.

The rumen, a diverticulum of the esophagus, is essentially a large fermentation vat in which different types of microorganisms actively break down the coarse fibrous material consumed by cattle and sheep. In the process of fermentation, gas is produced. To relieve the pressure caused by this normal production of gas, ruminants eruct or belch. Whenever an event or series of events restricts the ruminant's ability to eruct, gas pressures reach abnormal amounts in the rumen, thereby leading to overdistension, discomfort, and even death.

Bloat occurs in all domestic ruminants, but is most common in cattle grazed on a year-round basis, especially on pastures rich in alfalfa or the clovers. Bloat is not considered of economic importance in sheep in other countries, but is a serious economic aspect of sheep husbandry in the western United States.

Although pasture bloat may occur at any time, the incidence is highest in wet summers on rapidly growing clover-dominant pastures. Bloat occurs less often in animals in feedlots and barns.

Cause

Many complex factors have been implicated at one time or another as contributing to bloat in ruminants, and there are many different methods of classifying this condition; this discussion will classify the disease by nature of probable cause, that is, physical bloat, biochemical bloat, and hereditary bloat.

Hereditary Bloat

Hereditary bloat is commonly seen in dwarf cattle, and dwarf calves are habitual bloaters. A few of these individuals have been studied. These studies have found that anatomical defects natural to the animals interfere with the eructation process. Some families or strains seem to be more susceptible than others, and in this light, the condition appears to be inherited; however, the exact nature is undetermined. The bloat may be caused by an accumulation of factors on a given farm or property that may predispose the animals to the disease.

Physical Bloat

Physical bloat is a result of interference with the eructation reflex, which hinders the passage of gas. Any type of obstruction in the esophagus—foreign bodies, abscesses, adhesions, or gastritis—may predispose an animal to this condition. Overfilling of the rumen with feed and moisture to such an extent that the cardial orifice is obstructed, preventing the release of gas pressure, also leads to bloat.

Physical bloat may be caused by such solid objects as corncobs, turnips, apples, potatoes, or peaches, which commonly lodge in the esophagus and prevent eructation. External pressure on the esophagus by enlarged mediastinal lymph nodes or interference with cardial innervation, as in indigestion and diaphragmatic hernia (occurring sporadically in young calves), are further examples.

Biochemical Bloat

The overproduction of gas by microorganisms within the rumen, or anything of a chemical nature which has to do with destruction of the reflex action of the eructation process, leads to bloat. Overfeeding, damage to the right ventral branch of the vagus nerve, drugs and poisonous plants that bring about hypomotility of the rumen, and alkalosis, which may cause paralysis of the rumen, are all factors that have been implicated.

All types of bloat have one thing in common: the bloat results from a failure to get rid of fermentation gases as rapidly as they are formed. Overproduction of gas, per se, is not the important factor because normal animals can eliminate more gas than is normally produced under bloating conditions.

Factors Influencing Susceptibility

The occurrence of bloat varies with the location of and the type of management on a particular property. The season of the year is important with dairy cattle. Pasture bloat is most common in the spring and early summer, when cattle are grazing on succulent legumes, such as alfalfa and clover. In the feedlots, however, bloat is seen in the late summer and early fall, when cattle are brought in from pasture and fed fresh young hay. Alfalfa hay harvested in the fast-growing stage is particularly conducive to bloat.

Bloat is directly related to the consumption of diets high in legumes and concentrates. There appears to be no correlation between amount and rate of consumption of the forages. However, rations high in starch and protein are conducive to the production of excessive amounts of gas by the slime-producing bacteria residing in the rumen. A secondary factor is that animals put out to pasture on succulent feed often overgraze, thereby producing a moisture level in the rumen so high that it covers the cardial orifice of the esophagus and prevents the escape of gas.

Any circumstance that leads to an increase of alkalosis in the rumen may lead to paralysis of the rumen itself. The administration of alkali, either orally or intravenously, causes this condition; although reflex mechanisms are not eliminated, they are greatly weakened by the chemical.

Mechanical injury, obstruction of the esophagus, and reticulitis that results from ingesting hardware frequently lead to bloat. Abnormal growths in any area that may put pressure on the esophagus may lead to restriction of eructation and to bloat. However, the importance of such abnormalities appears to be minor.

Drugs and toxic factors produced by rumen microorganisms have been implicated as agents that reduce rumen motility and may interfere with eructation. Therefore, ingestion of legumes, which stimulate rumen microorganisms, may understandably result in bloat at one time or another. Other factors, e.g., overfilling of the stomach, may also be important in legume bloat. The relative importance of these factors is unknown, but is presumed to be minor compared to the effect of excess production of bubbles by the slime-producing bacteria within the rumen following consumption of legumes.

The bloat caused by legumes is primarily characterized by the production of froth; there is then little free gas within the rumen. Gas bubbles trapped in the ingesta create a situation resembling sticky foam

that does not allow the escape of the gas. Cows dying of bloat invariably have froth in the rumen. However, the rumen contents of animals that have been dead for several hours frequently contain only free gas because the froth breaks down after death.

Clinical Signs

Antemortem signs observed in bloated cattle include gaseous extension of the left flank and the abdomen, uneasiness as indicated by stamping of the feet, frequent urination and defecation, extension of the head and neck, labored breathing, slight protrusion of the tongue, and, finally, collapse and death without a struggle.

Death from bloat has been thought to be caused by mechanical interference with circulation and respiration from overdistension of the rumen. Biochemical alterations of plasma due to the abnormal absorption of carbon dioxide and other noxious gases produced in the rumen have also been implicated. Normally, carbon dioxide and methane gases are innocuous but, under pressure, may be forced into the capillary circulation, thus causing intoxication.

Postmortem Signs

The most prominent sign is distension of the rumen; however, this may be seen as a natural postmortem phenomenon in all ruminants because gas continues to be produced after death.

Generalized signs include extreme congestion of the lymphoid tissue of the head and neck, and absence of congestion in the muscles and lymph nodes of the hindquarters. Extensive hemorrhages into the mucosa of the trachea and congestion of large areas of the ventral sacs in the rumen may be found. Edema of connective tissue is not associated with lesions of muscle tissue. The rumen is filled to maximum capacity and overextended; it usually contains a mixture of feed and stable foam.

The upper plain contains a mass of free gas, but foam and feed fill the cardia. There is an absence of blood in the vessels and organs of the abdomen and the thoracic cavity (including the heart) although peripheral blood vessels are congested.

Diagnosis

The diagnosis of bloat is based on typical clinical signs and on the finding of froth in the rumen of dead animals suspected of bloat.

Treatment and Prevention

Bloat may be caused by one or more of a series of complicating conditions predisposing a ruminant animal to excessive gas production and the inability to relieve this condition by eructation. Because no single entity causes bloat in domestic animals, the condition must be controlled by careful application of management practices. However, these practices are subject to many inexplicable failures, and therefore, only guarded recommendations may be made. In general, procedures to attempt to control bloat include provision of adequate minerals, salt, and water in the diet (a nonbloating type of diet, obviously). Secondly, nonbloaters should be selected for breeding, and all dwarf animals should be eliminated from the breeding herd.

Pasturing should be controlled so that hungry animals do not overfeed on growing legumes. Wherever possible, animals grazing on legume pastures should be restricted to as much feed as they will consume in one day, requiring them to graze thoroughly. If possible, and wherever bloating becomes a problem in a given field, it may be well to spray the field with light mineral oils or peanut oil to reduce the frothy bloating. In some instances, antibiotics may be added to the feed of animals on high-concentrate diets; however, this provides only minimal protection and rapidly induces changes in the rumen flora. It may sometimes be efficacious to add surface-active agents, such as detergents, to ruminant feeds. If at all possible, straight legume pastures should be avoided. If animals are turned out on fast-growing young legume pastures, dry forage should be provided before they are allowed to graze.

When changing feeds becomes necessary, it is important to change slowly to prevent overeating. Green alfalfa should be chopped and mixed with straw so that the fresh alfalfa does not layer in the rumen, forcing the moisture level above the cardial orifice. Cattle will overeat when put on succulent pasture after a period of dry feeding.

When bloating occurs, treatment must be initiated immediately because animals suffering from bloat may die within 1 hour. The method of treatment varies with the degree of distension. If time permits, a stomach tube can be passed into the rumen to expel some of the gas. In more severe cases, however, a trocar can be passed into the rumen through the left paralumbar fossa to relieve the distension; however, this should be attempted only when death is imminent. A handful of common laundry detergent put into the mouth often brings about a reflex eructation, providing some relief for nonfrothy bloat and helping to lower the surface tension of froth (the gas consolidates into one large bubble). To prevent recurrences once bloat has been primarily relieved, stand animals with front quarters elevated, and if necessary, apply a stomach tube or a stick across the mouth to provide an open passageway for the relief of gas.

Development of medicated salts that may be left in fields and barns for free-choice consumption by ruminants has indicated that some measure of control may be possible.

Abomasal Displacement

The abomasum, the fourth or true stomach of ruminants, is subject to shifting in the abdomen of cattle. When its position is altered to the extent of blocking the entrance and exit of the abomasum, thus causing entrapment of the contents, the alteration of function of the digestive system causes clinical signs of disease. The disease primarily affects dairy cows but has occurred in both male and female calves and adults of all breeds.

As a disease of dairy cows, abomasal displacement occurs with sufficient frequency to be of economic significance. Affected cows may have a sudden decrease in milk production, become unproductive for the current lactation, or so severely affected that death results.

Cause

The causes of abomasal displacement are related to a loss of muscle tone and contractability of the abomasum. A reduced emptying rate ensues, gas accumulates, and the organ shifts position. The severity of clinical signs is directly related to the degree and the duration of blockage at the pylorus. The longer the condition persists, the greater the distention caused by entrapped contents and gas, and the more unfavorable the prognosis for recovery.

The disease occurs most frequently in the early postpartum period. Consequently, the space in the abdomen occupied by the gravid uterus may force a change in location of the abomasum. It has also been suggested that the contractions during parturition may initiate displacement.

Low roughage-high concentrate diets predispose animals to displacement. This is partly due to a lack of bulk in the rumen, but more to a drop in rumen pH resulting from decreased saliva and increased fermentation of carbohydrates. The result is atony of the abomasal wall and a decreased emptying rate, accumulation of gas, and displacement. Displacement of the abomasum from its normal location (on the abdominal floor and slightly to the right of the midline) can be to the left, under the rumen and between the rumen and left abdominal wall, or to the right, twisting upward on either a vertical or horizontal axis. The signs produced by displacement to the left are much less severe because incarceration is not complete; thus some movement of digestive contents is allowed. Signs produced by right displacement vary according to the degree of twisting or torsion.

Frequently, abomasal displacement occurs either concurrent with or subsequent to the stress of other severe systemic diseases, such as mastitis. The stress of severe systemic diseases is also linked to the loss of tone and contractability of the abomasum that results from general digestive-tract stasis.

Signs

Early signs of left abomasal displacement are depressed appetite and milk production; normal rectal temperature, respiration rate, and pulse rate; mild ketonuria; scant but normal feces; and slight distention of the left abdomen. Examination of the left abdomen by auscultation and percussion may give evidence of a gas-filled viscus between the rumen and the left abdominal wall. If displacement is allowed to continue for several days, the loss of appetite is reflected in loss of weight as well as in reduction of milk produced. The cow may become toxic and dehydrated from the development of metabolic alkalosis. The dehydration and toxicity cause a sunken appearance to the eyes, dry, inelastic skin, and dark-red mucous membranes.

Signs of right displacement vary. They may be similar to signs of early left displacement or to those resulting from severe toxicity and dehydration. The right abdomen is distended and sounds of gas and fluid may be found by percussion and auscultation of the right abdomen. If distention of the abomasum is sufficient, it can be palpated through the rectum.

Diagnosis

Diagnosis is based on the history of sudden onset, its proximity to calving time, the type of feed, and clinical signs. Definite diagnosis may require differentiating the signs from those produced by other diseases and by special tests. A positive diagnosis can be obtained by performing an exploratory laparotomy, which is considered practical if the surgical approach is made on a site providing access to repair. The disease must be differentiated from ketosis, traumatic gastritis, indigestion or rumen acidosis, cecal torsion, and intestinal obstruction.

Prevention

Sudden changes in diet are a potential cause of any digestive disturbance. Animals that are pushed to their limits in regard to converting feed to milk or meat are particularly susceptible to digestive disease resulting from either rapid change or unbalanced rations. Unbalanced rations commonly cause abomasal displacement. High-producing dairy cows respond to high-energy rations with increases in milk production. The attempt to increase consumption of concentrated high-energy feeds at the expense of bulky roughage increases the incidence of abomasal displacement.

Therefore, prevention can be accomplished by increasing the intake of hay or coarse roughage in proportion to concentrate. A 50/50 dry matter ratio is recommended as the safest; the ratio should never exceed 40/60 roughage to grain concentrate. Dairymen often attempt to adhere to this ratio by offering a free choice of hay in addition to a high-energy lactating ration. This is successful for the cows opting for the hay, but is ineffective for those ignoring the choice. The safest way to bunk feed a complete diet is to mix chopped hay (4 to 6 inches long) with the ration to assure an intake of approximately 5 pounds per day.

Early lush grass pastures and high moisture silage increase the incidence of displacement. Again, prevention can be accomplished by adding hay to the daily ration.

Treatment

Correction of the condition can be accomplished in a variety of ways, including running the animal around a pasture, giving the animal a bouncy ride in a truck or trailer, rolling the cow on her back, administering medicine, or surgically reducing and fixating the abomasum. All methods may prove successful under certain conditions. Running, bouncing, or rolling may relieve the gas pressure and restore the organ to its proper place. Medical therapy may also produce relief.

However, there is a high percentage of recurrence of the condition without surgical correction. Estimates are that 80% of displacements will recur unless the organ is replaced and sutured in its proper location. Even with surgical correction, the condition may require supportive fluids and drug therapy to restore the cow. In some instances, especially when the organ is twisted on the right side, nerve damage prevents recovery.

There are a number of different approaches to surgical fixation. All have advantages and disadvantages and are generally successful.

Traumatic Gastritis of Cattle (Hardware Disease)

According to the disease classification in Chapter 1, the name of this disease infers that it is a violent injury to the stomach (gastric) of cattle. Because cattle have several stomachs and the one affected in this disease is the reticulum, the disease is also called traumatic reticulitis. Whatever its name, the disease is the result of the cattle swallowing an object that falls into the reticulum, penetrates it, and causes a variety of signs. The major effect of the injury is loss of appetite and subsequent loss of condition.

The object swallowed can be any of a number of items—nails, pieces of wire, screws, bolts, slivers of glass, large needles, or any object that is heavy and sharp. Because most commercial feeds are screened with magnets to remove such material, the incidence of the disease has diminished in recent years. However, pastures can contain such objects, hay fields

may be located around construction sites, or metal can be deposited accidentally in feed bunks. A ruminant of any age is susceptible to this possibility, but because of their eating habits, adult cattle seem to be affected more often.

Cattle are not discriminating about what they swallow. They use their tongue and lips to pick up their feed, chew it enough to add saliva, and swallow a large amount at a time. Their esophagus is large and tough and ends in a groove between the rumen and reticulum (Fig. 2–1). The heavier material drops into the bottom of the reticulum. The reticulum regularly contracts during the process of rumination and while moving ingesta through the digestive system. If the object is caught in the folds of the lining of the reticulum, it could easily penetrate the lining during contraction. The actual penetration probably causes some pain—like getting a sli-

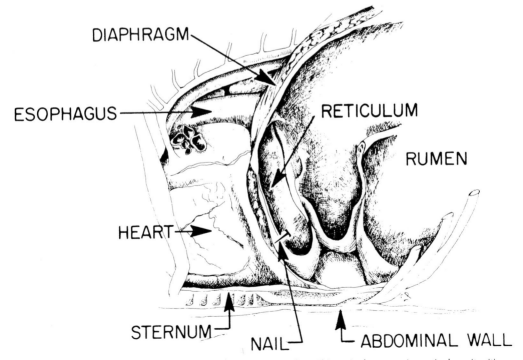

Fig. 2–1. Diagram showing potential point of penetration of a nail in reticulum, causing reticuloperitonitis.

ver in a finger—but the reaction of creating a hole in the wall and seepage of stomach contents through the hole causes severe pain. The pain is the result of the infection and inflammation on the outside of the reticulum. The effect is like stapling the bottom of the reticulum to the abdominal wall. The reticulum can no longer move freely, and if it does move, it is painful. The immediate response of the animal is to stop eating.

After the initial reaction to the penetration of a foreign object, the animal may resume eating, but not heartily, after a few days. There are several possibilities for the progress of the disease after the initial penetration:

1. An acute generalized peritonitis could develop.

2. A local abscess could develop.

3. The offending object could migrate forward through the diaphragm and cause a pleural abscess.

4. The object could penetrate the diaphragm and the pericardium (heart sac).

5. The object could migrate in another direction to involve the omasum, abomasum, or liver.

6. The object could migrate to the outside through the skin.

Signs

The signs of the disease vary according to when the disease is first noticed. If noticed at the time of initial penetration, the animal will be off feed, have an increase in body temperature, have slowed rumen contractions, will be reluctant to move, may stand with arched back to relieve pain, may grunt when breathing or moving, and will be sensitive to pressure over the area of the reticulum. If a generalized peritonitis develops, the animal will not eat, will develop a diarrhea, have a high temperature, become progressively weaker, and eventually die. If a localized infection is the sole result, the cow may return to eating, temperature will return to near normal, and the cow will appear to be losing weight gradually: milk production

will be reduced, but there will be no acute signs. Other signs that develop depend on where the object migrates. If it causes a pleural abscess or an abscess around the heart, there will be signs of respiratory and circulation changes. Ultimately, in this situation, the jugular veins become distended, there may be edema or fluid in the tissues in the brisket area, and fluid sounds may be heard around the heart and lungs.

Diagnosis

The diagnosis of traumatic gastritis is based on a history of possible objects being ingested and the signs listed previously. Experienced diagnosticians usually have their own method for detecting pain. Because cattle tolerate pain differently, it is not always a consistent sign. Other means of collecting signs include the use of test puncture to detect the presence of an abscess, analysis of blood to detect the presence of an infection, and the use of a metal detector to determine the possible location of the object. The use of a metal detector is questionable because it fails to detect glass or plastic. Radiographs of this area can be taken if facilities are available. However, most veterinarians find it quicker and less expensive to perform an exploratory operation to examine directly the area involved.

Prevention

Prevention measures are obvious—removal of all potentially offending material from the diet of the cattle. There are reports of some success from placing magnets in the reticulum of all cattle potentially exposed. Supposedly, the metal would collect around the magnet and would not penetrate.

Treatment

Treatment is successful in the very early stages of the disease. If the disease is diagnosed before the object has completely migrated through the reticulum, surgical removal of the object is successful. Another approach during the early stages is to place the animal on an inclined plane so that the animal stands with its front end elevated for a week or more. This has the effect of pulling the reticulum away from the diaphragm. Another method is to place a magnet in the reticulum by having the animal swallow it. The magnet may pull the object back inside the reticulum. Radical surgery on advanced cases of pleural abscesses or pericarditis is sometimes successful.

Equine Colic

Equine colic is not an infectious contagious disease of extreme economic importance to food animal production. However, colic is a common term and generally is understood to mean abdominal pain caused by some sort of digestive upset. Applied to horses, colic can be mild with transient pain of no consequence or acute with excruciating pain literally causing a horse to violently self-destruct. Obviously there is a wide range of causes and resulting diseases that produce such a contrast in signs.

Abdominal pain is usually derived from some alteration in the digestive system. The source, however, could be from the reproductive or urinary system, and diagnosis requires differentiation. A brief discussion of equine digestion and the anatomy of the system may help to understand the potential for disease and the signs produced.

Horses are herbivorous and are capable of digesting grasses or hay and grains. Lips and incisor teeth are used to pick up feed for mastication. The cheek teeth or molars are used to grind the feed as saliva softens and lubricates. Missing teeth, sharp points, or infections in the mouth that could make mastication painful or incomplete may result in the swallowing of dry, coarse feed. This could cause difficulty in passage of feed through the esophagus (blockage of esophagus or choke) or impair normal digestion in the stomach (impaction). Ingesta usually moves fairly rapidly through the stomach after mixing with gastric juices and passes through the small intestine for selective absorption. At the junction of the small intestine and colon, a large diverticulum (cecum) provides further breakdown of ingesta by bacterial action. The ingesta moves through a series of loops and turns into the colon eventually to pass out of the rectum at the anus. The normal appearance and consistency of the residue (feces) after fluids, electrolytes, and nutrients are absorbed is a formed bolus or ball of undigested fibrous material. The color of feces depends on the original feed; for example, feces may range from bright green if the horse is grazing new pasture to light brown if the horse is eating well-cured, dry hay.

Much can occur along the route from the mouth to the anus to cause disease and pain. Blockage at any point causes distention of the tract in front of the blockage. Horses do not eruct or vomit safely; therefore, accumulations of gas or fluids must traverse the tract. Blockage can occur for a variety of reasons:

1. As mentioned earlier, the ingesta could lack the moisture or lubrication needed to move it along.

2. The tubular gut may not have the normal peristaltic wavelike contractions necessary to move the ingesta.

3. Excessive gas could be produced by fermentation, causing excessive dilatation.

4. Peristaltic waves in the gut wall could be so vigorous that they cause a telescoping of the tubular intestine.

5. The loops of intestine could become twisted and cause complete blockage.

6. Adhesions with other organs in the abdomen may limit movement or strangulate intestines.

7. Loops of intestine may be displaced and strangulate through attaching mesentery.

Signs

To provide relief from any of the above conditions, the nature of the disorder and its cause must be determined. Horses are quite honest in showing pain, but do not necessarily indicate where it is located. One of the first signs of abdominal pain is a general uneasiness or restlessness. Stomping of the feet or pawing or kicking at the belly may be an indication of abdominal discomfort. An anxious expression in the eyes and intermittent turning of the head toward the abdomen usually indicates a "colicky" pain. Frequent intervals of lying down, getting up, and lying down and rolling usually are a pointed indication. Frequent apparent attempts to urinate or defecate by stretching and raising the tail are a sign of abdominal pain. As pain increases, the signs may become more exaggerated, sweating occurs, and pulse rate increases.

Diagnosis

Diagnosis requires an evaluation of the history (perhaps a rapid change in diet or exhaustion from overwork) and the signs exhibited. In addition to the behavioral signs shown by the animal, the digestive tract must be closely examined from beginning to end. Oral examination and passage of a stomach tube provide information regarding areas up to and including the stomach. Reflux of fluid from the stomach usually indicates blockage at the pylorus or in the small intestine. Auscultation of the abdomen by stethoscope may indicate the absence or presence of gas. Rectal palpation may indicate the area of obstruction. A sterile aspiration of the abdomen by hypodermic needle for peritoneal fluid aids in determining the status of any intestinal damage. Occasionally, when general signs are unfavorable and diagnosis is still uncertain, surgical exploration of the abdomen may be necessary for a positive diagnosis.

Treatment

A tentative diagnosis should be obtained before any treatment is given. However, because of the acuteness of pain and the potential for further damage, administration of drugs for relief from pain may be necessary before diagnosis is made. Mild flatulent colic may be relieved by giving mineral oil and an antiferment by stomach tube. Often, walking (not trotting) and time are sufficient to relieve the source of pain. Passage of gas and feces from the rectum is a welcome sight during an episode of "colic." Lack of response to sedation or mineral oil with continuation of or increase in signs is an indication for surgical intervention. The decision is difficult because it must be made early for surgery to be successful.

Regardless of the cause for colic, if the general condition of the horse indicates potential endotoxemia as a result of indigestion, fluids and electrolytes must be given to sustain life. In addition, administration of drugs may be necessary to combat shock.

Prevention

Most equine colic can be prevented by careful management. Some general rules are:

1. Do not make radical changes in diet, and do not allow access to unlimited grain.

2. Have teeth examined and treated if necessary to insure thorough mastication of feed.

3. Worm the horse on a regular schedule to avoid damage by intestinal or stomach worms or larvae.

4. Do not work the horse hard after feeding.

5. Do not allow unlimited access to water immediately after exercise.

Hemorrhagic Enterotoxemia

Hemorrhagic enterotoxemia is an acute disease of young calves, sheep, goats, cattle, and pigs. It is characterized by sudden onset, a profuse hemorrhagic enteritis, and sudden death. The disease is seasonal, with the greatest incidence occurring in late winter and early spring.

Historically, this disease was first described in 1930 in England as a disease of adult sheep in an area limited to the Romney marsh area. It was called "struck" in that country because of the rapidity of the development of symptoms and subsequent death. More recently, it has been studied in sheep and cattle in the western part of the United States and has been isolated from an outbreak in pigs in Minnesota.

Cause

Hemorrhagic enterotoxemia is caused by Clostridium perfringens type C toxin. The beta toxin of type C organisms is inactivated by trypsin, and this fact probably explains why the enterotoxemia is largely restricted to young, suckling animals. Type C is one of six antigenic types of C. perfringens, and beta toxin produced by type C is the most potent of all these toxins. Toxin is produced in the intestine because of the favorable conditions for the growth of the organisms produced by enteritis; this is associated with overfeeding and results in intestinal stasis, which rapidly favors the absorption of the toxin.

Transmission

Transmission of the C. perfringens organism is universal. The organism is a common soil contaminant and a normal part of the flora of the intestinal tract of most animals. The susceptible hosts are calves under 2 weeks of age, piglets under 1 week, adult sheep and goats, and, occasionally, adult cattle. The factor influenc-ing susceptibility is enteritis from overeating or some other cause, resulting in stasis of the intestinal tract. Stasis allows for absorption of greater-than-normal amounts of toxin, with the rapid production of signs.

Clinical Signs

Type C intoxication of hemorrhagic enterotoxemia is usually fatal to vigorous suckling calves under 2 weeks of age and piglets under 1 week of age. It is characterized by sudden onset, hemorrhagic enteritis, bloody diarrhea, and early death. Affected calves are commonly from dams that are heavy milk producers. Unfavorable, inclement weather at calving time is believed to have some influence on the incidence and severity of the disease. The disease also occurs in lambs and pigs under similar conditions. In pigs, the signs usually appear on the first or second day after birth; the heaviest mortality occurs on the second through the fifth day. The morbidity within litters varies and ranges from a single pig per litter to the entire litter. Most commonly, however, only some of the affected litters die. Diarrhea is consistently observed, except in animals with peracute cases. Such animals suddenly collapse and die before the onset of diarrhea. In acute cases, most piglets die on the first or second postnatal day, and bright red, watery feces are evident. Animals with a subacute clinical course of the disease of 2 to 3 days' duration have reddish brown liquid feces, whereas animals that have the disease for a slightly longer duration have colorless, liquid feces in which particles of gray, necrotic debris may be seen.

Commonly, the syndrome is a fatal, nonhemorrhagic, diarrheal disease of several days' duration; recovery is rare. In calves, the most common signs are listlessness, weakness, and failure to nurse, accompanied by evidence of colicky pains, such as kicking at the abdomen or uneasiness and rolling from side to side. A hemorrhagic diarrhea is evident after the other signs appear. There is rapid progression of the signs through prostration, tetanic spasms, and early death. The normal course of the disease in calves varies from 2 to 24 hours, and in many instances, the animals die without demonstrating overt signs. The temperature remains normal to subnormal. Mild cases do occur; upon recovery, these animals fail to make normal gains but have a good antitoxin titer.

Postmortem Signs

Postmortem lesions are usually noted to be hemorrhagic in character. The prominent lesion is a necrotic, hemorrhagic enterocolitis. The lumen of the intestine is filled with blood and tissue debris. Small hemorrhages occur on the thymus, the heart, and the covering of the intestinal tract.

The lymph nodes show an appreciable degree of swelling, and there are small pinpoint hemorrhages on the thymus gland and on the diaphragm. The heart sac contains an excess of fluid with some clotting, and the third stomach (in the case of calves) is distended with partially coagulated milk. The membranes of the stomach are inflamed and covered with a thick, tenacious, mucoid membrane. There may be areas of local necrosis throughout the intestinal tract.

Diagnosis

Diagnosis in the field is made on the history of sudden death in calves under 2 weeks of age and pigs under 1 week of age. Supportive diagnosis is made on postmortem signs. However, positive diagnosis is confirmed only by demonstration of the type C toxin in the intestinal contents and by isolation of the C. perfringens organisms from scrapings of the intestinal walls. The veterinarian can advise as to the method of preserving the intestinal content for transmission to a diagnostic laboratory.

Prevention

Hemorrhagic enterotoxemia can best be controlled by vaccination of the breeding herd of cattle with type C toxoid. It is recommended that 2 doses be administered, 4 weeks apart, the first year; booster doses should be given annually. Vaccination of dams confers passive immunity to the offspring, via the colostrum, that lasts 3 to 5 weeks. Calves from nonimmunized dams can be immunized with antitoxin soon after birth. Cows should be immunized with the toxoid 2 to 4 months prior to parturition, with a booster injection administered 3 to 5 weeks following the first injection.

In sows, a similar course should be followed. Because of the sudden onset and rapid course in piglets, it is usually not considered profitable to vaccinate baby pigs; they must obtain passive immunity from the sow through the colostrum.

Hog Cholera

Since it was first reported in 1830, hog cholera has been a highly contagious virus disease of swine causing almost 100% mortality. Before it was eradicated from the United States, annual cost estimates to the swine industry were approximately 50 million dollars. Even though this disease is no longer an economic threat to the swine industry, it is worthy of some discussion in this text as a classic example of animal disease control.

The geographic distribution of hog cholera has been worldwide. The virus is transmitted by direct contact, congenital infection, such vectors as flies, lung-worms, fomite, chronic carriers, and un-cooked pork garbage. The virus is patho-genic for swine only. The swine producers of the United States virtually "lived" with the disease for more than a century until a concerted effort was made to eradicate it in the 1960s. The disease was controlled by immunization using various types of vac-cines. Although effective, the widespread use of simultaneous serum and live virus innoculations probably helped to perpet-uate the disease as a result of careless han-dling of the vaccine.

Signs

The signs of disease are most often acute, occurring 2 to 6 days following ex-posure. A temperature of 105° F or more and a loss of appetite and activity may be the first signs. The disease may run a rapid course, with death occurring as early as 24 to 48 hours following initial signs. Ne-cropsy findings from pigs that died rapidly are so minimal that the disease has been described as "lesionless." Pigs surviving for longer periods characteristically huddle together, refuse to eat, but may drink wa-ter if forced to move (Fig. 2–2). Although constipated initially, a light brown, watery diarrhea develops. Other signs include a sticky exudate in the corner of the eye, purple to red splotches on the skin, and, occasionally, terminal convulsions. Pigs

surviving to a chronic status have lived as long as 95 days.

Although the swine industry existed in the face of the threat of this disease, there was extensive study to determine diagnos-tic features and control of transmission. Characteristic blood and tissue changes had been determined, as had tests for the presence of the virus. Despite uncertainty as to the exact nature of the existence of the virus outside swine, the Animal Health Division of the USDA decided eradication of the disease was possible.

Hog cholera had been successfully elimi-nated from Canada and Great Britain, and U.S. pork was losing export markets. The United States Livestock Sanitary Associ-ation proposed a four-phase program, which was adopted by the USDA in 1962. This program, which was revised in 1964, was considered successful when, in 1974, the United States had received no reports of the disease for almost 1 year. The salient parts of the original program were:

Phase I. Preparation by dissemination of information about the program, surveys to determine incidence, standardized diag-nostic tests, and enforcement of garbage feeding and quarantine laws.

Phase II. Reduction of incidence by quarantining infected and exposed hogs, stopping interstate movement of infected hogs, and supervising the interstate move-ment of all swine.

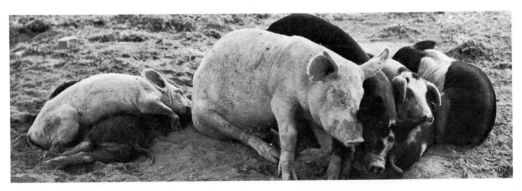

Fig. 2–2. A distressing photograph of young hogs suffering from hog cholera huddled in a characteristic manner in the barnyard.

Phase III.   Elimination of outbreaks by depopulation and control of vaccines.

Phase IV.   Protection against reinfection by establishing restrictions on the movement of all swine.

The success of this program was basically the result of removing the virus by eliminating the infected host. By stopping movement of any swine surrounding an outbreak, the potential transmission was eliminated. Prompt diagnosis, reporting of outbreaks, and destruction of infected pigs were encouraged by payment of indemnity. Elimination of all vaccinations prevented the possibility of changes in vaccines contributing to continuance of the disease.

Many people closely associated with the swine industry were skeptical of the prospects for success of this program. Credit for success belongs to those who had the foresight to develop the program and to the scientists who gathered the diagnostic tools and epidemiologic information. The result has been more efficient production of pork and elimination of waste of resources.

Chapter 3

Diseases with Signs of Nervous System Changes

Diseases other than those covered in this chapter, such as rabies, encephelomyelitis, and milk fever, cause nervous signs. Poisonous substances such as strychnine, chlorinated hydrocarbons, and organic phosphates also cause nervous signs. The diseases selected for this chapter are common and need to be differentiated from others causing signs of alteration of the nervous system.

RECOMMENDED READING

Amstutz, HE: Bovine Medicine and Surgery. 2nd Edition. Chaps. 4 and 11. Santa Barbara, CA, American Veterinary Publications, 1980.
Blood, DC, Henderson, JA, and Radostits, OM: Veterinary Medicine: A Textbook of the Diseases of Cattle, Sheep, Pigs and Horses. 5th Edition. Philadelphia, Lea & Febiger, 1974.
Jensen, R: Diseases of Sheep. Chaps. 2, 4, 6. Philadelphia, Lea & Febiger, 1974.

Tetanus

Tetanus, or lockjaw, results from a wound infection of deep tissue with Clostridium tetani. It is characterized by intoxication accompanied by spasmodic and tonic contractions of voluntary muscles. All common types of livestock, except poultry, are susceptible to tetanus. A list of the more highly susceptible animals includes men, horses, mules, sheep, and goats. Swine are more obviously susceptible when young because the highest percentage of cases occurs at an early age; however, this may be at least partly due to the greater opportunity for infection at that time because of the practice of clipping needle teeth. The distribution of the disease is essentially worldwide, but it occurs most commonly in old farming areas with large livestock populations and where manure is commonly returned to the land. Tetanus occurs more often in tropical and subtropical regions than in the colder parts of the world.

C. tetani and the disease it produces are of historical interest. The disease has been known and greatly feared for centuries. As early as the fourth century B.C. physicians believed tetanus was caused by the wind. In 1884, scientists produced tetanus in a rabbit by using materials from a person who had died of lockjaw. It was shown that toxins produced by C. tetani would produce the disease when injected into rabbits. Later it was shown that immunization against the toxins could be obtained by the injection of small doses of blood serum from experimentally infected animals. Such a serum could neutralize the toxin both in vitro and in vivo. Thus, it was in connection with tetanus that (1) anaerobic techniques were first used, (2) bacterial toxins were first demonstrated, and (3) the foundation for serum therapy was first laid.

CAUSE

Tetanus is caused by the toxins of C. tetani. The vegetative form of the organism is a slender, gram-positive, anaerobic rod. Spores are usually terminal in location and 2 to 3 times the diameter of the vegetative rods, giving the sporulated rod the appearance of a spoon or drumstick when seen microscopically.

C. tetani is commonly found in the soil and in the feces of most animals. The spores are resistant, especially when protected from light and extremes of heat, and exist almost indefinitely in the soil.

As are other clostridial species, this microorganism is anaerobic and finds suitable conditions for growth in deep wounds, where two toxins are produced by the growing bacteria. One of the toxins is a hemolysin and of slight importance in producing the signs of the disease. The other, however, is a neurotoxin that causes the characteristic signs of tetanus.

TRANSMISSION

C. tetani gains entrance to the body via wounds. The disease commonly results from deep, penetrating, or puncture wounds in which there is considerable tissue damage and gross contamination by soil or manure. Probably the most common port of entry in lambs, calves, and pigs is via castration wounds. Occasionally, the infection gains entrance into the body at the unhealed navel shortly after birth, via the dental alveoli during eruption of teeth, or possibly through wounds caused by unclipped needle teeth. In a small number of instances, no likely portal of infection can be demonstrated; these are often referred to as idiopathic tetanus. Some such cases probably result from infection of small wounds that heal before tetanus appears.

Adult animals often acquire the infection through parturition wounds, dental caries, wire cuts, nail stab wounds, shearing cuts, dehorning wounds, castration, or any number of traumatic experiences.

SIGNS

The incubation period for tetanus is from 1 to 3 weeks following infection. The first sign is a mild muscle stiffness, which may be localized but is more often general. The progress of the disease is generally rapid enough, however, that the signs are distinctive within 24 to 36 hours. The characteristic manifestation, from which the disease is named, is that of tonic or tetanic muscle spasms. Although all muscles are affected, the stronger muscles overcome the weaker or opposing muscles and produce the attitudes characteristic of the disease. The contraction of the muscles of the back, neck, and tail produce orthotonos and even opisthotonos; contraction of the muscles of the limbs produces a sawhorse attitude (the extensor muscles are stronger than the flexors); and contraction of the muscles of mastication causes lockjaw (Fig. 3-1). Difficulty in locomotion may be demonstrated first in turning or backing, but the animal soon finds that walking or even standing is difficult. Pigs often show unusual erectness of the ears, and all animals exhibit some protrusion of the third eyelid. Spasms of the muscles of respiration permit only shallow and therefore rapid breathing. A fast heart rate may be quite noticeable. Animals often fall to the ground with head thrown back and all muscles rigid.

As the disease progresses, the animals become apprehensive and sensitive to sensory stimuli. Sudden movements, sharp noises, or slaps intensify muscle spasms or protrusions of the third eyelid. Toward the end of a fatal attack, the temperature may

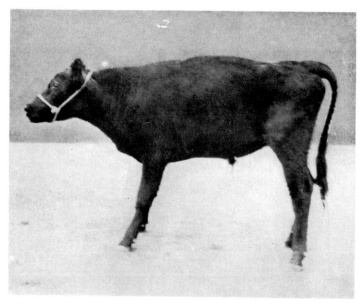

Fig. 3–1. Tetanus following castration. Sawhorse attitude, extended head and neck, and raised tail are all apparent. (From Gibbons, WJ: Clinical Diagnosis of Diseases of Large Animals. Philadelphia, Lea & Febiger, 1966.)

increase to 108 to 110° F. The disease is almost always generalized and fatal, especially in very young animals. The mortality averages 80% among adults. There is a prolonged convalescent period for those that recover. Death is undoubtedly due to anoxia from interference with respiratory and cardiac functions.

PATHOGENESIS

Under favorable conditions, the spores carried into the wound become vegetative, multiplying and forming toxins at the original site. The toxin includes tetanolysin, a hemolytic portion, and tetanospasmin, the more important lethal fraction. Tetanus toxin is one of the most poisonous substances known. The organisms show little tendency to spread to other parts of the body. However, the toxin apparently passes by diffusion into the surrounding medium, into the blood, and then spreads into the central nervous system.

The incubation period for tetanus is usually 1 to 3 weeks but occasionally is shorter or much longer. The length of the incubation period is probably influenced not only by the number of infecting organisms but by the conditions set up in the contaminated wound, particularly by the amount of tissue damage incurred. Washed spores of the tetanus organism do not germinate when injected into healthy tissue, presumably because the oxygen tension is too high in such tissue. However, if a culture that also contains toxin is injected, germination does occur and the disease results. Likewise, the disease occurs with regularity when washed spores are introduced with some irritant solution. Thus, tetanus spores apparently germinate only in dead or injured tissues, or those altered in a way resulting in lowered oxygen tension. In addition, tetanus toxin adversely affects leukocytes and thus interferes with phagocytosis of the spores.

Rigor mortis appears rapidly following death from tetanus. However, no significant gross lesions are characteristic for this disease. The blood is usually dark red and may be poorly clotted. Pulmonary congestion and edema may be noticeable, and a few hemorrhages may be found in the serous membranes of the chest cavity. Necrosis at the site of injury may be so slight that it is unnoticed.

DIAGNOSIS

Despite the fact that there are no characteristic gross lesions in tetanus, the diagnosis usually presents no particular difficulty. The signs are not likely to be confused with those of any other diseases except strychnine poisoning, eclampsia, lead poisoning, or rabies. However, the last three diseases have additional signs that should easily clear up any confusion. Signs of tetanus are often accompanied by a history of recent castration or the presence of a contaminated or infected wound. Therefore, clinical diagnosis is based on history and signs. Tetanus is confirmed at autopsy by the absence of significant gross lesions and, if the infected wound can be demonstrated, by the presence of the characteristic bacteria. It is seldom necessary to go beyond the clinical examination to establish the diagnosis of tetanus.

PREVENTION

There is no practical means of eliminating the spores of C. tetani from the environment. Losses from tetanus, though generally sporadic, may be enzootic because of heavy concentrations of spores in the soil.

There are three points at which attempts can be made to break the cycle of the disease:

1. Because tetanus is a wound-infection disease, every effort should be made to prevent unnecessary wounds by removing from the environment any sharp objects, such as bare nail points, wire, splinters, broken glass, or projecting boards. Swine producers must clip the sharp points from the needle teeth of newborn pigs.

2. A clean environment should be provided so far as possible; that is, maternity pens should be periodically sanitized and

kept as free of manure as possible and umbilical cords should be treated with antiseptic soon after birth. Castration, dehorning, and docking operations should be performed with every reasonable precaution to prevent infection.

3. When conditions of exposure cannot be controlled or when the species is very susceptible (e.g., horses, man), immunization is practical and effective.

Temporary passive immunity is provided by administration of antitoxin. A dose of 1500 to 3000 units of antitoxin is routinely administered to horses that receive any type of wound. Use of antitoxin in conjunction with treatment of wounds in other species depends on the type of wound and the degree of environmental risk in relation to the value of the animal.

The development of active immunity in horses and valuable animals of other species is both practical and essential. Active immunity is developed by a series of 2 or 3 injections of tetanus toxoid at intervals of about 1 month. These injections are reinforced by an annual booster.

TREATMENT

Treatment of tetanus after signs have developed may be impractical for lambs or pigs because of the cost in nursing care and medicine. However, animals can be maintained under sedation and force fed while undergoing antibiotic therapy. Large doses of antitoxin are considered a valuable adjunct to a course of treatment. Affected animals must be housed and isolated from external stimuli.

Enterotoxemia

Enterotoxemia (overeating disease, pulpy kidney disease) is an acute, highly fatal poisoning of sheep, principally lambs, caused by absorption of a toxin produced by the bacterium Clostridium perfringens, type D. The toxin is produced in the intestinal tract; the condition is therefore an autointoxication. Enterotoxemia is characterized by cerebral symptoms, convulsions, sudden prostration, and death. Adult animals are less susceptible to enterotoxemia, and the condition is most often seen in young, fat, fast-growing, greedy lambs in feedlots or on pastures. It has been very costly to the sheep industry around the world. However, effective control has evolved from good management practices and the use of biologic products for immunization against the toxin.

Geographically, enterotoxemia is found wherever sheep are raised. Historically, the organism that causes enterotoxemia was first isolated and described at Johns Hopkins University from a decomposing human cadaver before the turn of the cen-

tury. Since that time, Bacillus perfringens, as it was first called, has been isolated from a variety of conditions and has been given several names. For many years, the bacterium was known as Clostridium welchii; however, by universal agreement, it is now called Clostridium perfringens and further is designated by toxogenic type, as each type of toxin causes a different set of symptoms in different species of animals.

CAUSE

Clostridium perfringens is a large, anaerobically cultured, nonmotile, encapsulated, hemolytic, gas-producing, rod-shaped organism capable of producing at least six types of powerful toxins that are designated by letters of the alphabet. These endotoxins contain 15 antigenic toxic fractions. Each is immunogenically distinct from the others and has been designated by a small Greek letter. Several conditions in livestock are produced by C. perfringens. Usually, one fraction is present in quantity along with minor amounts of the other toxins in each specific disease entity.

Type A.   Type A was first isolated from man, and although it has been reported in lambs and calves, it is relatively unimportant from the veterinary point of view. Type A is found in the intestinal tract of most warm-blooded species.

Type B.   The toxins produced by type B C. perfringens cause a condition known as lamb dysentery. This condition has been reported also in colts and in calves but is primarily seen in very young lambs.

Type C.   This type affects sheep, goats, cattle, and pigs. It was reported in England as a condition called "struck" in sheep, and it causes hemorrhagic enterotoxemia of lambs, calves, and baby pigs in this country.

Type D.   This type is the cause of a common and destructive disease of sheep, calves, and goats, and has been described in all sheep-raising parts of the world. It is known variously as enterotoxemia, pulpy kidney disease, and overeating disease. Type D has been isolated from lambs, sheep, calves, and cattle.

Type E.   Type E C. perfringens causes dysentery and enterotoxemia in lambs and calves but is of little importance from the veterinary point of view.

Type F.   This type causes a chronic enteritis in man. It is believed that the ability to produce toxic signs in livestock is related to the ability of the organism to produce high levels of hyaluronidase, which is linked with the pathogenicity of the toxins.

TRANSMISSION

The predisposing cause of intoxication with C. perfringens type D is overeating or gorging on highly nutritive feed ingredients; this causes a disturbance in the digestive tract and creates an ideal environment for the multiplication of the organism. This organism is commonly present in the stomach and intestinal tract in normal warm-blooded animals and is found in the soil in all parts of the world. The immediate cause of the disease is the absorption into the blood of a toxin liberated by the bacterium. The organism is worldwide in distribution and affects sheep of all ages, goats, and calves. It occurs in all seasons of the year under widely different types of husbandry.

The intoxication is perhaps most common in lambs 2 to 6 weeks of age and in weaned lambs in the feedlot or on lush, green pasture. Enterotoxemia frequently affects the most vigorous, fast-growing lambs in the flock. Outbreaks are commonly associated with an increase in feed availability or with a change in type of feed.

FACTORS INFLUENCING SUSCEPTIBILITY

Although the prominent role of type D toxin is generally recognized, the circumstances allowing rapid proliferation of the organism in the intestinal tract are not clearly understood. One common factor seems to be the ingestion of extensive amounts of feed that is high in carbohydrates, as undigested starch granules are frequently found in the intestinal contents of acutely affected lambs. Digestive disturbances associated with sudden changes in diet and with the transition to solid food by nursing lambs may be other factors. The intoxication is most often seen in the fattest, greediest lambs in the flock. In nursing lambs, the condition occurs when the ewes are on good pastures of grass, winter wheat, or early spring alfalfa; among feeder lambs on rich clover pastures or in feedlots with a heavy grain ration, the most greedy eaters suddenly die. This occurrence is directly related to management procedures, as many feeders are willing to sacrifice a number of animals to increase the growth rate of most of the animals in the feedlot.

When enterotoxemia is seen in mature sheep, it is usually associated with the management practice of turning sheep into corn fields or excessively lush pastures during extremely hot weather.

CLINICAL SIGNS

Lambs affected with C. perfringens type D toxin usually do not exhibit visible signs. The disease may be acute; the animal can be found dead in the morning after having been in good condition the previous night. The first indication of the disease is sudden death in the best-conditioned animals. When signs are noticed, they appear a few hours before death. Lambs may suddenly jump, fall to the ground in a convulsive seizure, and die. Others show signs of irritability, indicating an inflammation of the brain. Such signs as circling, pushing against fixed objects, or mental depression are often seen in the early stages of the disease. Lambs showing convulsions may have only a slight rise in temperature. In less acute cases, diarrhea may develop with recovery occurring in a few of the lambs. In these instances, loss of appetite, depression, vomiting, and paralysis, followed by diarrhea, which may persist for several days, bring about a rapid loss of weight with slow recovery.

POSTMORTEM SIGNS

C. perfringens type D bacteria are normally present in the intestinal tract of all mammals and are abundantly found in the soil. Because of the acute nature of the toxemia, this condition must be differentiated from other infectious diseases causing sudden death in livestock. As C. perfringens type D organisms are found in the intestinal tracts of most animals dying of acute symptoms, they are frequently found as postmortem invaders from the intestinal tract into the tissues of bloating animals. For this reason, some caution is necessary when drawing conclusions based on the presence of the organism in tissues collected after death. Clostridium perfringens type D is found more often than any other organism in the so-called gas gangrene infections; however, it is generally associated with other species of

anaerobes in this process. When a young lamb overeats, atony of the intestinal tract provides the proper anaerobic environmental conditions for the rapid growth of C. perfringens and the proliferation of the type D toxin. As the organism multiplies, it rapidly produces the toxin. Because of the atony of the small intestine, the toxin then is absorbed into the blood, and the signs and lesions listed above are rapidly produced. Because rapid death is one of the prominent signs of this condition, postmortem lesions are of relatively little importance in animals dying in the peracute stage. However, several postmortem signs are readily attributable to this intoxication. When a lamb is opened immediately upon death, there is usually little to be seen in the kidneys. However, the synonym "pulpy kidney disease" has often been attributed to this condition because 3 or 4 hours after death the kidneys appear swollen, dark red, soft, and mushy, with a consistency of strawberry jam. This is not a constant lesion however and is only seen in animals that have been dead for several hours before autopsy is attempted. There is passive congestion of the lungs and the trachea. There is an increase in the fluid in the heart sac, and it is often coagulated. Diffuse hemorrhages, occasionally large blotches but most often small dot-like hemorrhages, occur on all the intestinal organs, abdominal muscles, the diaphragm, and the thymus gland. The livers of animals dead for several hours appear friable, dark, and congested; they are occasionally spotted with light-colored areas 2 to 4 mm in diameter. The urinary bladder is usually empty, and there is frequently an absence of solids or fluids in the intestinal tract but much food in the stomach.

DIAGNOSIS

Diagnosis in the field is usually based on sudden death in young, fat, vigorous, greedy lambs. However, because death occurs suddenly in other diseases, an autopsy must be performed. Specimens taken by a veterinarian and sent to a laboratory should include urine and intestinal contents for confirmation of the type D toxin.

PREVENTION

Enterotoxemia is difficult to treat because death is rapid. However, the control of enterotoxemia may be effected by proper husbandry and by immunization. The method of control depends on the type of husbandry followed by the farmer or rancher. Grain rations should be reduced when the disease first appears and then gradually increased as the outbreak subsides. Sometimes losses can be minimized by carefully sorting lambs as to size and space at the feed trough to prevent the greedy lambs from overeating. Grazing stock should be moved temporarily to other types of feed. Under range conditions, the movement of lambs is not feasible; therefore, supplemental feeding of well-cured alfalfa is helpful in some instances. Sudden changes in type and amount of feed should always be avoided because such changes tend to create overeating. When an outbreak does occur, type D antitoxin, which confers a temporary immunity, may be used to control the outbreak. However, losses in lambs younger than about 6 weeks of age cannot be controlled in this fashion. The protection for such lambs is best accomplished by immunizing the ewes with 2 doses of C. perfringens type D toxoid; the second dose is given about 2 weeks before lambing. The passive immunity conferred on the lambs lasts about 6 weeks; afterward, the lamb itself may then be vaccinated. The first injection can be conveniently given at the time of docking. To provide effective protection, 2 doses separated by an interval of not less than 4 weeks are usually regarded as necessary. Immunity following the first injection takes about 10 days to develop, whereas that following the second injection not only is stronger but develops more quickly. Six months after the second injection, a booster dose is sometimes necessary. Antitoxin gives an immediate immunity lasting 2 to 3 weeks. It is used to stop death losses in lambs following an outbreak of enterotoxemia and may also be used to immunize feedlot lambs on a short-term feeding basis for as many as 3 weeks.

Toxoid is intended to stimulate the development in healthy animals of an immunity lasting 5 or 6 months; protective immunity requires 10 days to develop. Toxoid, therefore, should be administered at least 10 days before sheep are placed on full feed. There may be a reaction in the tissues at the site of injection. Because this reaction may persist for at least 30 days, toxoid should not be used if the animals are intended for slaughter within that time. Toxoid should not be injected into lambs under 2 months of age.

Antitoxin and toxoid should not be injected at the same time because the immediate immunity established by the antitoxin prevents the body tissues from reacting to the toxoid. The antitoxin or toxoid is injected by aseptic means usually under the skin of the fleece-free area in back of the place where the foreleg joins the body. Injections at this site help to prevent unnecessary lameness.

Ketosis

Ketosis is a metabolic disease of lactating cows caused by an imbalance between nutritive intake and nutritive requirements. The disease occurs within a few days or weeks after calving. It is characterized by low blood-glucose levels, depletion of liver-glucose stores, mobilization of body proteins as amino acids, mobilization and utilization of fat storage depots of the body, and infiltration of the liver, associated with increased production of ketone bodies in the blood and urine.

An accurate appraisal of the economic loss caused by ketosis is difficult because the disease is not associated with high mortality. Observations from widely separated areas indicate that clinical ketosis is responsible for a heavy loss in milk production. It also is of considerable importance to the beef cattle industry, as it occurs frequently in the heavier milking cows of the beef breeds. Ketosis in cattle occurs in practically every country in which dairying is practiced. However, only a few cases occur in areas where modern selection and production management practices are ignored. Therefore, ketosis is apparently a disease associated with high production of both calves and milk.

Ketosis may occur at all ages, but it is most common during the years of greatest production, that is, after the second or third lactation. Therefore, it is associated with age and sex of dairy animals.

CAUSE

Although several predisposing factors are associated with ketosis, the exact cause is not known. A complex of factors can be associated with this metabolic condition. It may be said with certainty, however, that interactions between the diet and endocrine glands in cattle are mechanisms of development of the disease. Certain aspects of ruminant physiology and nutrition predispose the lactating dairy cow to ketosis. Metabolic dependence on rumen microorganisms and the excessive demands of heavy lactation are principal contributing factors. Competition by the mammary gland for energy products leads to a metabolic breakdown. When the major energy mechanism is blocked, the ruminant cannot effectively utilize certain substances produced by digestion, among them ketone bodies (or acids). Consequently, the incidence of clinical ketosis can be minimized by bringing nutrient consumption into line with physiologic needs, particularly in the critical pre- and postpartum periods.

One school of thought regards the disease primarily as a carbohydrate deficiency associated with a defect in carbohydrate metabolism. Another theory is that the disease is basically a temporary adrenal insufficiency.

The carbohydrate-deficiency hypothesis is based on the observation that little of the various forms of carbohydrate ingested by the ruminant is absorbed as glucose. If this is so, the lactating cow receives little or no carbohydrate beyond that required for the synthesis of the lactose secreted in the milk. The metabolic-defect theory is supported by the fact that ketosis occurs when the dietary intake of carbohydrate or its precursors is inadequate. As only a few lactating cows develop ketosis, there is obviously some deviation in the metabolism of affected animals. This metabolic defect remains undiscovered, but since the endocrine glands influence the function of the various biochemical pathways, the defect may be caused by some endocrine imbalance.

When all available evidence is evaluated, it is difficult to escape the conclusion that carbohydrate deficiency, and not adrenal insufficiency, is of major importance in the cause of ketosis in cattle. Any evidence of adrenal insufficiency appears to support and strengthen the carbohydrate-deficiency concept.

FACTORS INFLUENCING SUSCEPTIBILITY

At the time of calving and lactation, an animal's nutritive and metabolic requirements are increased about 100%—partly because of the loss of sugar, proteins, and fat in the milk and partly because of the increased metabolic work associated with the production and secretion of milk. If the dietary intake is adequate, the animal remains normal. If the diet cannot maintain approximate normal levels of blood glucose and liver glycogen, an imbalance in metabolism occurs.

This upset is indicated by anorexia, hypoglycemia, and depletion of liver glycogen. In response to these disturbances, compensatory metabolic adjustments are initiated in an attempt to correct the imbalance. When the blood-glucose level is low, the carbohydrate stores in the liver tend to become depleted in an attempt to maintain the level of blood glucose and, in turn, the carbohydrate requirements of other tissues. Ketosis tends to develop under these conditions.

There are several classifications of ketosis, all of which have similar symptoms, although slight variations do occur. *Primary ketosis* indicates a simple imbalance between nutritive intake and nutritive requirements of lactating animals. *Secondary ketosis* may occur in varying intensities in lactating or non-lactating cattle and incudes instances in which the metabolic disturbance is precipitated or aggravated by infections, exposure, foreign bodies in the rumen, traumatic gastritis, peritonitis, mastitis, cystic ovaries, vaginitis, displacement of the abomasum, indigestion, and starvation.

Ketosis may also be classified as lactation ketosis, digestive ketosis, or nervous ketosis, depending on the premonitory symptoms. The first two types are similar in their manifestations. Nervous ketosis is evidenced by a derangement of the nervous system brought about by the temporary malnutrition of the brain caused by low blood-glucose levels. The condition can be described as a semiconscious state indicating a depression of the cortical nerve centers of the brain.

SIGNS

The signs of ketosis usually appear within 6 weeks following calving, especially in high-producing cows. All animals with uncomplicated ketosis do not have the same signs. Some show extreme nervousness and convulsions. Others may have a lack of appetite and constipation, with hard mucus-covered feces retained in the rectum. There may be a striking picture of depression accompanied by rapid weight loss, drop in milk production, staggering gait, and, finally, paralysis, with cattle lying with their heads tucked into the flank (in such instances, the disease resembles milk fever).

The body temperature and the respiratory and pulse rate are usually normal except in the nervous type, or when the ketosis is complicated by other conditions. However, as the severity of the condition varies directly with the degree of nutrient imbalance, animals may show shallow and increased respiration accompanied by a strong acetonic odor of the breath. Grinding of the teeth and some salivation may also occur.

Nervous signs in a small number of cases of ketosis are sometimes mistaken for signs attributed to rabies. Cows often push against the wall or stanchion, evidence unusual movements, and may even attack the handler. They usually hold their heads in a lowered position and appear blind. Lowered blood-glucose levels and high ketone levels in blood and urine are always present. Unless laboratory tests are made, the blood ketone levels will be difficult to demonstrate. However, simple chemical tests can be conducted on small samples of urine in the field; color changes indicate the level of ketone bodies in the urine.

Postmortem lesions of animals that have died as a result of fulminating ketosis are rather indistinct. Few gross changes may be seen, except that the liver may show a diffuse yellow color due to fatty infiltration. This liver change and the history of the animal prior to death present a presumptive diagnosis of ketosis.

PREVENTION

Ketosis, with or without complications, increases the metabolic requirements roughly in proportion to the magnitude of the combined stresses associated with lactation and other disturbances.

Diet during pregnancy or lactation can

increase or reduce the chances of ketosis. If the diet consists entirely of roughage, fermentation in the rumen favors production of acetic acid; this cannot be converted to glucose but can form ketones. However, if the diet contains a high ratio of grains and concentrates, rumen fermentation favors production of propionic acid, which can be converted to glucose.

Animals susceptible to ketosis should be maintained on a relatively high-energy diet before calving, and the level should be increased substantially after parturition. To limit the degree of stress, one should take precautions to avoid marked changes in the environment of the animal during the parturient period.

TREATMENT

Treatment for primary ketosis is directed toward raising the level of blood glucose. This can be accomplished by intravenous injection of glucose, oral administration of sodium proprionate or propylene glycol, or administration of corticosteroids or ACTH. Response to treatment may be rapid and spectacular, but relapses requiring repeated treatment can occur. Sometimes response is poor, requiring continuous intravenous glucose and supportive therapy.

Toxemia of Pregnancy

Toxemia of pregnancy is a metabolic disease of sheep resembling ketosis in cattle. The disease is characterized by nervous involvement brought on by low blood sugar and depletion of liver glycogen.

Pregnancy toxemia occurs primarily among ewes in the last few weeks of gestation. Ewes carrying twins or triplets are particularly liable to the disease, although wethers and rams on starvation diets may develop the symptoms.

This disease is frequently found in range flocks where severe climatic conditions restrict grazing and where sheep are maintained at a poor level of nutrition for the latter part of pregnancy. Therefore, the disease is found worldwide.

CAUSE

The knowledge of the cause and pathogenesis of this disease is not complete. From critical observations, however, toxemia of pregnancy is apparently associated with stress and nutrition level. The primary cause of the toxemia is poor nutrition in late pregnancy. Ewes in good condition but carrying twins are more susceptible to this disease than are ewes carrying a single lamb or those in poor condition. The usual course of events follows a pattern: Ewes well fed at the beginning of pregnancy become overfat, suffer a setback in nutrition followed by a period of stress, and then die. Ewes on a high plane of nutrition die quickly when forced either to consume a poor-quality diet or to starve for a few days because of severe weather or mismanagement.

SIGNS

Affected ewes are not easily detected in the early stages of the disease. If the flock is driven, however, the affected ewes tend to fall behind, and, if closely examined, may exhibit a stilted gait with the head held high and often a slight tremor of the muscles of the face and lips. Later the animals become dull, appear blind although the eyes seem normal, and stand sleepily in one position with the head drooped, inattentive to their surroundings. Finally, they lie down, often with the head resting in the flank, and are unable to stand when assisted to their feet. Unconsciousness follows, and death occurs in 1 to 5 days.

Affected ewes generally show little or no change in level of blood calcium and do not respond to treatment by injections of calcium. The level of blood sugar is reduced, and ketones are present in the blood and urine in abnormal quantities. Similar changes can be caused in normal pregnant ewes by starving them for a time, and conditions that cause a setback late in pregnancy are likely to cause an outbreak. Malnutrition during the later stages of pregnancy, especially if associated with cold wet weather, is a predisposing cause for losses in lean seasons.

Ewes left undisturbed on good grazing can die of pregnancy toxemia, but in such instances, some unknown factor causes them to lose appetite and, consequently, weight, in spite of the abundant feed.

At postmortem examination, the only striking feature (aside from the usual presence of two lambs in the uterus) is that the liver is soft and fatty and yellow to grayish-red in color.

DIAGNOSIS

Pregnancy toxemia is easily confused with milk fever or hypocalcemia. Many ewes are lost each season when they are mistakenly diagnosed as suffering from pregnancy toxemia. In fact, they are suffering from milk fever and could be saved by injections of calcium. With milk fever the signs occur just before or just after lambing; the course of the illness is short, and death occurs within 24 hours.

TREATMENT

Once signs have developed, the chance of recovery with any treatment known at present is slight. Occasionally, good results are obtained in early stages of the disease by drenching with molasses; however, this treatment appears to have no effect in other outbreaks.

Once toxemia is discovered, immediate steps should be taken to prevent more cases from developing. The flock should be given the best and most palatable feed available; if young nutritious hay is available, they should feed on it an hour or two every day. If the disease develops in a flock on good feed and in high condition, gentle exercise each day is beneficial; they should be taken at an easy pace for about 2 miles a day, and allowed to graze as they go. Ewes and lambs should be removed as they drop to facilitate the handling of the remainder. If individual ewes are of high value, the veterinarian may remove the lambs by cesarean section; if near term, the lambs as well as the dam may survive.

PREVENTION

Because treatment of pregnancy disease is of little value in the advanced stages, prevention is the best policy. It matters little if ewes lose weight slightly just after the mating period, but from the second month of pregnancy onward, they should be kept in good condition and should increase in weight. During the last 5 or 6 weeks of pregnancy, the lamb in the uterus achieves 80% of its total growth, and the ewe is also preparing for milk production when the lamb is born. The strain on the mother's resources is thus great, especially if she is carrying more than one lamb. Anything that lowers nutrition level at this time must be avoided as far as possible.

Ewes must be given the best feed and shelter available and a good and easily accessible water supply. If it is necessary to yard them during this period, good nutritious diet should be furnished with as little delay as possible. Do not change suddenly from one type of feed to another, but make the change gradually over a period of a few days. Failure to do so has frequently precipitated outbreaks of the disease.

In dry seasons, when natural feed is scarce, supplementary feeding of the breeding flock should be started while there is still plenty of roughage in the fields. The supplemental feed should be rich in easily digestible protein. Where natural protein-rich fodders, such as legumes, are available, a cereal supplement of corn, oats, or wheat may be fed. Alfalfa hay of good quality cannot be excelled.

It is impossible to recommend the quantity of supplement to feed under every condition. Overstocking, severe winter or summer conditions, and unseasonable cold wet weather may upset the most careful plans. Adequate reserves of hay and/or silage should be carried from year to year to allow for such possibilities.

Obesity should be prevented early in pregnancy, but an adequate, nutritious diet is particularly important during the last 6 weeks.

Botulism

Botulism is a fatal disease caused by the toxin of Clostridium botulinum and characterized by rapidly progressive motor paralysis. Botulism is not a bacterial infection, but rather is an intoxication caused by the ingestion of a preformed toxin, usually in decomposed or "spoiled" animal or vegetable matter. As a disease of man, judging by ancient edicts warning against their consumption, botulism was first ascribed to the eating of blood sausages. The peculiar form of neuroparalysis liable to follow the eating of such sausages was first accurately described in Wurthemberg in 1735; the actual term *botulismus* or sausage poisoning appeared in the medical literature of southern Germany about 150 years ago.

Botulism has been recognized as a disease of domestic animals since 1917, when it was first noted in horses. Veterinarians were quick to point out the striking similarity of botulism in man, limber neck in chickens, and forage poisoning in horses. Upon observation, it became evident that at least some of the outbreaks diagnosed as forage poisoning in horses were actually caused by C. botulinum. Of course, other outbreaks undoubtedly were encephalitis of viral origin.

Botulism in other species seems to occur relatively infrequently. This is due, in part, to species resistance to the toxin and also perhaps to other factors, such as eating habits. For example, outbreaks in cattle have been caused by feeding on carrion, as a result of perversion of appetite caused by mineral deficiency. In any event, cattle, sheep, swine, dogs, and cats are commonly regarded as relatively resistant to botulism. Wild ducks are susceptible, and large numbers have died from the disease. The disease has been reported in captive mink and the common laboratory animals. Guinea pigs and mice are susceptible and are the animals used to demonstrate the disease experimentally. Botulism as a naturally occurring disease in swine is now of no great importance because of modern feeding practices. However, C. botulinum is widely distributed in nature; it is found in soils, especially those well fertilized with animal wastes, and in fruits, vegetables, decaying organic matter, aquatic and emerging vegetation, and moldy hay.

CAUSE

The organism responsible for the production of the toxin that causes botulism is generally referred to as C. botulinum. On the basis of its proteolytic abilities, it is now commonly subdivided into two groups and designated as either C. botulinum (nonproteolytic) or C. para-botulinum (proteolytic). However, for purposes of general reference, both groups will be referred to collectively here as C. botulinum.

C. botulinum is a motile, gram-positive, rod-shaped bacterium occurring singly or in short chains. Spores are generally terminal or subterminal. Growth requires strict anaerobic conditions, such as those found in necrotic or decaying organic matter. Growth occurs within a wide range of temperatures including body temperatures, but is perhaps optimal at about 90°F. C. botulinum is commonly found in the soil and in the intestinal tract of healthy animals, where it causes no harm. But once the animal dies, the bacteria multiply rapidly and produce the toxin that causes intoxication when consumed by another animal.

TRANSMISSION

Because botulism is fundamentally an intoxication rather than an infection, it is not transmissible from animal to animal in the usual sense. This is true in spite of the fact that massive doses of toxin-free spores may rarely result in sufficient germination, multiplication, and toxin liberation, in vivo, to produce the disease. Several types of botulism toxin have been described, as have some subtypes. Variation in cultural features does not appear to be closely related to the type of toxin produced; that is, type B may be formed by proteolytic or nonproteolytic strains, whereas in either proteolytic or nonproteolytic strains, more than one type of toxin may be formed.

Even though the toxin is said to resist a degree of acidity equivalent to that of the gastric juice and to be impervious to the action of pepsin or trypsin, some animals are particularly resistant to oral doses of the toxin. This resistance may be due to slight absorption of the toxin through the small intestine of these animals. Further, the bacterial flora within the intestine may have a deleterious effect on the toxin.

FACTORS INFLUENCING SUSCEPTIBILITY

Botulism is rarely seen in livestock in the United States; in fact, it is more often seen in man than in animals. However, the intoxication may be seen in cattle, sheep, horses, and chickens. Swine are resistant to the condition.

In areas with a phosphorus deficiency, cattle and sheep may chew on the bones of dead animals in whose carcasses C. botulinum has multiplied and produced toxin, thereby incurring botulism. Forage poisoning of cattle and horses is due to botulism toxin that has developed on decaying silage and hay. Thus, starvation, mineral deficiencies, or any other factor associated with the ingestion of toxin-contaminated material predispose an animal to the condition.

CLINICAL SIGNS

Naturally and artificially affected animals appear to be affected in the same way. After the latent period of 8 to 72 hours, a progressive weakness of the voluntary muscles appears, usually beginning in the head and neck regions and spreading backward over the body. The weakness, leading to paralysis, is evidenced in the disturbance of several functions. The most obvious, of course, is the disturbance of locomotion. Weakness in the forelegs often appears first, followed by involvement of the hindlegs and, ultimately, by prostration caused by complete paralysis of all limbs. The muscles of the throat are often affected, resulting in inability to swallow and in excess salivation. The ears may droop more than usual, adding to the appearance of depression. Vision may be impaired. Superficial reflexes appear to be affected only in that motor responses become progressively weaker. The activity of smooth muscle is not affected, and the chief effect upon the circulatory system is a fast and uneven pulse. Ultimate involvement of the respiratory muscles results in cyanosis, anoxia, coma, and finally death from asphyxia. Animals that survive botulism may require weeks or even months for complete restoration to normal health.

POSTMORTEM SIGNS

Few postmortem lesions are noted other than infrequent hemorrhages in the lungs and the general signs associated with high temperature. There may be froth in the trachea, but this is not a common sign.

DIAGNOSIS

Diagnosis of botulism is generally based on history, signs, absence of gross lesions, and laboratory diagnosis of the offending toxin. Occasionally, the source of toxin can be demonstrated in the stomach of animals dead from the intoxication. For example, the eating of carrion can sometimes be determined at necropsy by noting the presence of maggots in the gut. When this occurs, it may lead to the source of the intoxication.

C. botulinum occasionally may be isolated from animals with botulism, but not with sufficient regularity to be of much value as a diagnostic procedure. Therefore, negative results do not preclude the possibility of botulism.

TREATMENT AND CONTROL

Although the toxins of C. botulinum are immunogenic, they may be used to produce not only antitoxin but also toxoids. To be of value in the prevention of botulism in animals, antitoxin must be used early in the course of the disease. The use of such products in swine is not practical, even in garbage-feeding enterprises, because of cost and the low incidence of the disease, which, in turn, is apparently the result of the natural resistance of swine to botulism. Cattle and sheep raised in phosphorus-deficient areas, however, can be immunized by the use of polyvalent toxoid. For best results, cattle and sheep should be vaccinated each spring before they are turned out on pasture or range.

Spoiled canned goods, spoiled garbage, and carrion appear to be the most frequently incriminated media in which botulism toxin is formed. Thus, in spite of the fact that swine are known to be relatively resistant to the action of the toxin, they should not knowingly be fed such products. Any food considered unfit for human consumption should not be fed to animals; this should be considered the first step in preventing botulism. The toxins are thermolabile; consequently, boiling of garbage for 30 minutes should destroy the toxins. The spores, on the other hand, have great thermal resistance, which apparently varies with the strain, the pH, and other conditions of the medium. The botulism spores survive for considerable lengths of time under dry heat, and freezing has little effect on either spores or toxin.

In view of the ubiquity of C. botulinum and its ability to survive under most natural conditions, there seems to be little hope of completely eradicating botulism. On the other hand, the disease should be found only under uncontrollable circumstances.

Hypomagnesemia

Hypomagnesemia, or grass tetany, is a metabolic disease of sheep and cattle of any age or condition, particularly beef cattle grazing on low-quality feed and subjected to climatic stress. The disease is most common, however, in lactating cows and ewes grazing on lush grass pastures in the spring.

Grass tetany is characterized by low blood-serum magnesium. However, it appears to be a mineral imbalance involving not only magnesium but also calcium and phosphorus. The disease occurs in Europe, Australia, New Zealand, North America, and other parts of the world where advanced animal husbandry and pasture methods are employed. The incidence varies from property to property, according to the type of management exercised, and this may account for the erroneous belief that the condition is of genetic origin.

CAUSE

The exact cause and the resulting pathogenesis of grass tetany are not well understood, although several predisposing factors have been associated with the disease.

Rapidly developing signs during the first few days after being turned out on grass pasture in the spring is a common history.

Hypomagnesemia occurs in mature cattle, usually over 4 years of age, when they have been maintained on low nutrition and then subjected to stress, such as cold, inclement weather, parturition, or movement. Agronomists have demonstrated that grasses grow quickly following a cold spell and that rapidly growing grasses are low in magnesium. Also, in the early spring in mixed pastures, grasses grow more quickly than do legumes, and the latter normally contain more magnesium than do grasses. In addition, the early, rapidly growing grasses are high in nitrogen, especially if the fields have been fertilized. All these factors contribute to lowered magnesium consumption and utilization.

Livestock grazed on wheat and other cereal grains (especially crested wheat grass) that provide a high intake of potassium develop a relative hypomagnesemia leading to clinical signs. Although other grasses are undoubtedly capable of causing grass tetany, crested wheat may be incriminated most frequently because it develops early in the spring and is ready for grazing before most other grasses.

Grass tetany appears to be more a result of low utilization of magnesium consumed than of low intake of magnesium. The fact that many pastures producing grass tetany have marginal levels of magnesium, with respect to animal requirements, compounds the problem and accelerates the development of the deficiency.

SIGNS

Signs of grass tetany are excitement, incoordination, loss of appetite, viciousness, staggering and falling, muscle twitching, anxious wild look, grinding of teeth, unusual salivation, general muscle contractions, labored breathing, and pounding heart beat. These signs are usually followed by convulsions and death.

There are two apparent types of grass tetany, acute and chronic. The acute type is characterized by sudden onset. The animal may be found dead shortly after being turned out to graze on lush grass, or, if observed, may suddenly appear frenzied, stagger, fall down into a convulsion and either die or recover, only to repeat the performance at short intervals until death occurs. In less acute cases the seizures may be 2 or 3 days apart but progress dramatically unless treated.

The chronic type can be diagnosed only by an examination of blood that reveals a lowering level of magnesium. However acute signs may develop whenever such an animal becomes stressed. During the chronic period, animals may lose weight but signs of hyperexcitability do not occur unless the serum magnesium levels drop below 1.0 mg per 100 ml. A drop in serum calcium is usually associated with the drop in magnesium. Cows affected by the chronic type of hypomagnesemia continue to eat and lactate, although milk production decreases.

Increased heart rate and loudness of heart sounds are diagnostic features of both types.

Hypomagnesemia may occur in calves maintained on a milk diet for 3 or 4 months. The condition is characterized by tetany, the same as seen in adults.

PREVENTION

Good management is essential in preventing this disease. Cows and ewes should be protected from the elements and maintained on a nutritious diet, especially during the last part of pregnancy.

The University of Illinois Extension Service recommends that "...herds with a current or recent history of grass tetany be fed supplemental magnesium. This is such an acute disease in many herds that affected animals may not recover even when calcium magnesium gluconate is administered promptly after the animal becomes tetanic. Feeding grade magnesium oxide

(MgO) is recommended as an economical product in which the magnesium is readily available. Current recommendations are directed toward ensuring an intake of ½ to 1 ounce per cow per day from late fall until the spring pastures have 'hardened'. Emphasis must be placed upon the daily intake since body stores of magnesium are not readily available. The MgO may be fed with grain or on silage. In herds fed only hay or pasture, 10 to 15% MgO may be mixed with loose salt. If greater percentages are used, the salt intake may be depressed. In order for this method to be effective in preventing clinical grass tetany it is essential that the MgO-salt mixture be (1) the only source of salt, (2) always readily available, and (3) consumed by each animal daily.

"It is helpful to administer 2 ounces of MgO in a capsule to cows that are treated intravenously and also to feed cows MgO in grain or silage for 2 weeks or more to help prevent relapses."

CHAPTER 4

Diseases with Signs of Respiratory System Changes

The nasal passages, larynx, trachea, and lungs are the major structures of the respiratory system. Changes that interfere with the free passage of air to and from the lungs cause vital embarrassment. Man may create the optimal environment in which to cope with impaired respiratory function, but farm animals do not have the luxury of creating special facilities in which to exist. To be economically productive, farm animals must not be handicapped by impaired respiration. The diseases in this section are examples of viral and/or bacterial infection of all segments of the respiratory tract except the larynx. The Recommended Practices section is included because it represents a joint effort by the cattle industry and the veterinary profession to prevent and control bovine respiratory diseases in the cow-calf herd.

RECOMMENDED READING

Amstutz, HE: Bovine Medicine and Surgery. 2nd Edition. Chaps. 3 and 14. Santa Barbara, American Veterinary Publications Inc., 1980.
Blood, DC, Henderson, JA, and Radostits, OM: Veterinary Medicine: A Textbook of the Diseases of Cattle, Sheep, Pigs, and Horses. 5th Edition. Philadelphia, Lea & Febiger, 1979.
Leman, AD, et al.: Diseases of Swine. 5th Edition. Chap. 47. Ames, IA, Iowa State University Press, 1981.

Pneumonia of Calves

Calves develop pneumonia in a variety of circumstances and as a result of infection with various organisms. One pneumonia is a part of or follows neonatal diarrhea of calves. This pneumonia is sometimes called a pneumoenteritis syndrome. There is a viral pneumonia of calves (primarily housed as opposed to range calves) caused by the parainfluenza 3 virus. Another pneumonia is caused by bacterial complication of the viral pneumonia. Some pneumonias result from extension of viruses, such as IBR. Also, calves develop pneumonia as a sequel to any debilitating disease.

PNEUMONIA AND DIARRHEA

Neonatal diarrhea was described in Chapter 2 as causing excessive fluid loss and dehydration. Tissue dehydration is detrimental to a defense mechanism against respiratory infections. The normal lining of the trachea and bronchii consists of specialized epithelial cells with hairlike cilia. These hairlike projections create a reverse or outward current to expel foreign material and exudate from the lungs. If there is excessive fluid loss from tissue cells because of diarrhea, the cells of the lining of the trachea and bronchii are shrunken and cannot perform the function of removing exudate from the lungs. The result is the inability to repel infecting bacteria and the pooling of exudate in the lungs. For an already weakened calf, this result is often fatal.

Signs of pneumonia in a newborn calf that is already suffering from a severe diarrhea may be insufficient to attract attention. When the calf starts to recover from the diarrhea, it is usually noticed to be breathing rapidly and to have a temperature of 103 to 105° F. Appetite is poor, and the calf is dull and depressed. The muzzle may become dry, and a purulent nasal discharge develops. Unless signs of respiratory infection are noticed early, the calf usually dies.

Prevention is based on keeping the calf in a dry, well-ventilated area away from aerosol contact with other calves. Damp, poorly cleaned, and unventilated barns with a strong ammonia odor can cause respiratory infection even without the stress of dehydration and diarrhea. Also, because these are nursing calves, care must be taken to prevent inhalation of milk or electrolyte solutions. Nipples with large openings allow fluids to flow faster than calves can nurse, especially if the bucket or bottle is held too high above the calf's head.

Treatment for pneumonia must be combined with relieving the dehydration and correcting the fluid balance. Systemic antibiotics should be started at the first indication of pneumonia and continued for several days after apparent recovery. Expectorants to loosen exudate and stimulate coughing are also indicated. Although a variety of organisms could be involved, a broad-spectrum antibiotic should be used unless there is time to culture exudate.

VIRAL PNEUMONIA OR ENZOOTIC PNEUMONIA OF CALVES

The most common virus to cause pneumonia in young calves is parainfluenza 3. This virus is present in all countries, and 85% of adult cattle carry its antibodies. Maternal antibodies in colostrum give some protection but are either present for an insufficient time or incapable of defending against heavy exposure. Calves raised in a single building are most susceptible because of transmission by air. The disease is mild if uncomplicated and generally affects calves from 1 to 4 months of age.

SIGNS

Clinical signs after exposure run a course of 5 to 8 days. Lacrimation, conjunctivitis, increased mucoid nasal discharge, inappetence, and general malaise are observed. Uncomplicated parainfluenza infection is characterized as an upper respiratory infection of sudden onset, with a temperature ranging from 104 to 108° F. Early in the infection, many animals show an initial high fever with no other evidence of clinical illness. In some animals, the elevated temperature persists for 25 to 48 hours and may be followed by prompt recovery. Most animals remaining febrile for more than 2 days show anorexia and mild depression and develop a dry, hacking cough with a clear, serous discharge.

There is concurrent hyperemia of the upper nasal and conjunctival mucous membranes with a slight flow of tears from the medial canthus of the eyes. Animals not infected with secondary bacterial invaders or with other viral infections and not subjected to undue stress promptly recover. This initial syndrome can be duplicated experimentally with intranasal installation of nasal culture; however, all animals so inoculated do not contract the disease. It is felt that some stress factor must be present to produce parainfluenza routinely, as observed in the field.

An increase in respiration is a common clinical observation, and labored breathing is present in some cases. There appears to be no hypersalivation in uncomplicated cases, and diarrhea is not noted. Morbidity may reach 100%, although fatalities in uncomplicated cases are virtually nonexistent.

The temperature is monophasic and the early leukopenia is followed, in protracted cases, by a leukocytosis caused by secondary invaders. Because the infection is usually associated with stress and is of short duration, its importance rests with the fact that it lowers body resistance, thus complicating other diseases or allowing secondary bacterial invaders to produce serious disease and death losses.

DIAGNOSIS

Diagnosis can be confirmed by virus isolation and tissue culture inhibition study. Presumptive diagnosis can be made from history, clinical signs, and failure to isolate any causal bacterial pathogens. An acute or mild upper-respiratory infection of short duration with concurrent leukopenia and absence of other findings is suggestive of parainfluenza.

PREVENTION

Because the disease is so easily transmitted to susceptible calves by inhaling air contaminated by the virus exhaled by infected calves, healthy calves must be separated from infected calves. Ventilation and sanitation for housed calves must be sufficient to "keep the air clean." Calf barns are notorious for air heavy with an ammonia odor and dampness. Although direct draft should be avoided, it is preferable to poor ventilation. I and many others believe that calves are healthier when staked out and widely separated atop a well-drained hill than when kept in a barn.

A successful vaccine has been produced to protect young cattle against parainfluenza 3. The increase in hemagglutination-inhibition titers of vaccinated animals has proved the vaccine's effectiveness. Several inactivated virus vaccines are commercially available and can be used on young calves. Polyvalent vaccines including parainfluenza 3, IBR, and Pasteurella are also available.

Vaccines are recommended for the protection of healthy animals against the respiratory disease. Because maternal antibodies may persist in calves until 4 or 5 months of age, vaccination is particularly recommended at 2 or 3 weeks prior to weaning of beef calves.

TREATMENT

As with other viral diseases, there are no specific therapeutic agents. Antibiotics are of value only in preventing complications caused by secondary bacterial agents. Uncomplicated parainfluenza pneumonia is best treated by avoiding all possible stress.

Infectious Atrophic Rhinitis of Swine

Infectious atrophic rhinitis is a highly transmissible disease of swine that causes atrophy or distortion of the nasal turbinates. The disease occurs in swine in most areas of the world. It is estimated that 5 to 10% of all swine slaughtered in principal swine-producing areas of the United States have turbinate atrophy. Lesions produced by the disease are found primarily in pigs 2 to 5 months of age. Severely affected pigs are unthrifty and susceptible to respiratory infections. Although the disease has been described for more than 100 years and has been thoroughly investigated, its cause had not been clearly defined until the last decade.

CAUSE

In 1956, Switzer was able to reproduce the disease by instilling Bordetella bronchiseptica, which was recovered from atrophic swine turbinates, into the nasal passages of baby pigs. Also, there have been numerous reports throughout the years of finding Pasteurella multocida in the nasal passages of affected pigs. Bordetella bronchiseptica is generally accepted as the primary cause of infectious atrophic rhinitis in pigs in the United States. However, it is believed that both Pasteurella multocida and Bordetella bronchiseptica are the cause of the disease in swine in the Netherlands.

B. bronchiseptica can cause mild respiratory-tract infections in dogs, cats, rabbits, mice, turkeys, horses, and man, as well as in pigs.

TRANSMISSION

The organism is transmitted as an aerosol from infected to noninfected pigs. However, because the organism is so widely present in other species, infection could result from a source other than infected pigs. As infected animals get older, the infection may not produce clinical signs, but sows or boars may be carriers. Transmission from sows to their litter is considered a common method of perpetuating the disease in a herd.

Ideally, housing vacated by infected pigs should be fumigated and left idle for 3 months; however, it has been found that quarters vacated for only 2 weeks did not produce infection in susceptible pigs.

CLINICAL SIGNS

Sneezing and sniffling by baby pigs are an early indication of the disease. Sneezing is an attempt to remove exudate from the nasal passages. There are other causes of sneezing and rhinitis in pigs, but infectious atrophic rhinitis is the most common cause. As the disease progresses, there may be flecks of blood in the exudate produced by the sneezing. It is common to see an accumulation of dirt and moisture at the inner commissure of the eye resulting from excessive lacrimation.

Infected pigs do not grow as quickly as normal pigs. As the infected pigs grow, the face and nose may show changes indicating turbinate and bone damage. The frontal bones may not develop normally, causing a narrowing of the distance between the eyes. The nose may be turned to one side by as much as 45 degrees. If both nasal turbinates are atrophied equally, the snout may have a pushed-in appearance with wrinkled skin behind it. Because part of the defensive mechanism for protecting the respiratory system has been damaged, pigs with atrophied nasal turbinates often develop pneumonia.

POSTMORTEM SIGNS

The changes involve the nasal mucosa and the turbinate bones. The normal scroll-like pattern (Fig. 4–1) of the turbinates is altered in varying degrees when exposed by a cross-sectional cut behind the second cheek tooth. The ventral turbinate may be only slightly atrophied or the entire turbinate may be absent. The changes may be evident on one side only or both sides (Fig. 4–2). The mucous membranes of the turbinates, if present, may be covered with a mucopurulent exudate. The frontal sinuses may be small with an inflamed mucous membrane.

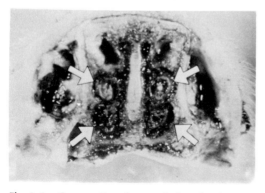

Fig. 4–1. Cross section of nares of a hog showing normal scroll-like pattern of turbinates.

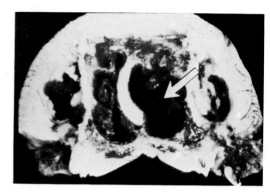

Fig. 4–2. Cross section of disrupted turbinates due to atrophic rhinitis.

DIAGNOSIS

The diagnosis for atrophic rhinitis is the key to controlling the disease. This disease plagued the swine industry for many years until the cause was finally established and the method of diagnosis devised. By submitting a percentage of a pig crop to examination of the turbinates at slaughter, a producer could monitor the incidence of infection in his herd. Since determining that Bordetella bronchiseptica is the primary cause, it has been possible to determine infection in the live pig.

After cleaning the nostrils, sterile swabs are introduced into the nasal passages to pick up exudate that contains the organism. These swabs are quickly cultured at a laboratory for presence of B. bronchiseptica. Swabbing and culturing only once with negative results is not considered more than 67% accurate. A total of three negative results obtained at weekly intervals is considered 95% accurate.

Clinical signs of sneezing and nasal distortion are highly significant. Culturing and finding the organism are diagnostic.

CONTROL AND PREVENTION

This disease was one of the reasons for the development of the Specific Pathogen Free (SPF) programs. It was considered necessary to completely break contact between baby pigs and the sow and the environment at birth. This was successful as a preventive measure and led to the development of disease-free herds. However, the problems of expense and difficulties of raising newborns without the benefit of the dam's colostrum were expensive.

Swine producers have approached the problem according to the value of their herds and the extent of their facilities. Some producers accept the presence of infection and suppress the clinical effects by adding antibiotics or sulfonamides to the feed. This adds cost but reduces losses for poor growth rates.

Some producers try to keep the disease minimized by continually culling pigs that show signs. This practice is unsatisfactory because infected pigs can carry and spread the disease without showing signs.

Another control method recommended is to house a sow separately with her pigs and not to allow any outside contacts for at least a month after weaning. Breeding stock is selected from pigs not showing signs.

Farrowing can be supervised to prevent pigs from getting near the head of the sow, to allow the pigs to nurse once, and then to remove and hand raise them.

The use of diagnostic swabbing of nasal passages can lead to clearing a herd of all infected animals. This process is long, but it is practical in valuable breeding herds.

1. Determine the status of the herd by examining for turbinate atrophy in a percentage of market pigs, and swab 4- to 10-week-old pigs for the organism. Subject the cultures to sensitivity tests for sulfonamides.

2. Retain old sows in preference to gilts because aged animals are more apt to have recovered from the disease.

3. Completely isolate the breeding herd from all other potentially infected pigs.

4. Using the results of the sensitivity tests in No. 1, medicate the feed or water with sulfonamides for 5 to 6 weeks.

5. Swab both sides of the nasal passages of all breeding animals at the end of the medication period. Remove all animals having positive swab cultures and retain only those having three negative swab cultures.

6. Swab and culture again 2 weeks before farrowing. The farrowing house should be cleaned, fumigated, and kept empty for 6 weeks before sows are allowed to enter.

A bacterin for B. bronchiseptica is being marketed, and there are reports of its effective use.

TREATMENT

Sulfonamides are effective for most strains of B. bronchiseptica. However, because some strains are resistant, sensitivity tests are necessary. Sulfamethazine in feed or sulfathiazole in drinking water for a period of 5 weeks clears the infection.

Infectious Bovine Rhinotracheitis

Infectious bovine rhinotracheitis (IBR), or rednose, is a viral disease of cattle, goats, and wild deer and is characterized by intense inflammation of the upper respiratory tract, the eyes, and the reproductive tract. Rednose is an acute, contagious infection that may be an important cause of abortion in both dairy and beef cattle. When it is complicated by secondary bacterial invaders, bronchopneumonia often results.

Rednose was recognized as a clinical entity in 1950 in dairies and feedlots in the western part of the United States. Since that time, the disease has been diagnosed in all parts of North America. Subsequently, the disease, in one or more of its forms, has been recognized and the virus isolated from cattle in all parts of the world except South America. Although the disease persisted at a low incidence in dairies, it became so common in the great feedlots of Colorado and California that it attracted more attention than any other disease of feedlot cattle. This attention has led to the rapid discovery of the cause of the disease and the development of an effective vaccine.

In early reports, the disease was characterized by an acute inflammation of the upper respiratory tract. Noticeable clinical signs were fiery red nose, copious nasal discharge, polypnea with open-mouth breathing, and fever.

CAUSE

Infectious bovine rhinotracheitis is caused by a filterable virus. The virus is fairly stable in a slightly alkaline environment at very low temperatures, but is less stable at room temperatures and does not remain viable for more than 3 days.

The virus is readily isolated from the nasal and ocular fluids of infected cattle, but rarely from blood. The virus may also be found in the tissues of aborted fetuses, in the placenta and vulval secretions of cows that abort, and in the brain of calves with encephalitis. It may also be found on the penis and prepuce of range bulls. Cattle that appear healthy may harbor the virus in the respiratory tract for several months, and so serve as healthy carriers of the disease.

The disease may occur in cattle of all ages and in both sexes, at any time, but the greatest incidence is found in the fall, when range cattle are concentrated in feedlots.

TRANSMISSION

The virus is primarily transmitted directly by infected droplets that are spread by coughing animals and by contact with infected secretions from the nose, eyes, and vulva. Secondarily, the infection is spread indirectly by contaminated examination instruments. The virus may invade the placenta and developing fetus by way of the maternal circulation, and consequently, either abortion or death and resorption of the fetus about 60 days after infection may occur. Young nursing calves may contract the infection from the dams and develop signs of encephalitis.

The usual method of spreading the virus to the vulva of cows and penis and prepuce of bulls is venereal. Within 36 to 48 hours following infection, clinical signs begin to appear.

All ages and all breeds of cattle are susceptible to the virus; however, range cattle seldom develop clinical signs of the disease until they are confined in fairly large groups. The incidence is highest and the course most severe in feedlot cattle because the virus becomes more virulent by passage through many susceptible animals.

FACTORS INFLUENCING SUSCEPTIBILITY

Upon primary infection with the respiratory form of rednose, the incidence of the disease and the virulence of the infection are both low in the first few animals in an affected herd. However, virulence is enhanced by continual passage through a herd. The respiratory form of the disease is most prevalent in large concentrations of animals, whereas the genital infection is more often seen in smaller breeding herds where passage is not sufficiently swift or continuous to enhance virulence. A mild infection may occur in heifers before breeding age, thereby making them immune to all forms of the disease; if these heifers subsequently breed with infected bulls, however, they may become carriers and shedders of the virus.

SIGNS

Rednose can exist in a mild or inapparent form. The incubation period is usually 5 to 7 days, but even in infected feedlots, 30 to 60 days may pass before clinical signs are observed in most animals. The temperature is usually high, with typical readings from 104 to 107° F. This sign is accompanied by a clear serous nasal discharge which may, on rare occasions, contain flecks of blood.

This discharge later becomes mucopurulent and tends to be tenacious, hanging in strands from a fiery red or encrusted muzzle (Fig. 4–3). It is accompanied by depression, lack of appetite, and labored breathing caused by accumulations of serofibrinous exudate in the trachea, sinuses, and turbinates. Coughing is a prominent sign, often accompanied by a heaving action with the tongue protruded. Primary pneumonia is not usually present, although at times, secondary bronchial pneumonia develops. Morbidity in infected herds may range from 25 to 100%; however, mortality is usually low, ranging from 0 to 5%.

Lacrimation due to conjunctivitis is commonly present, and close observation reveals edema and small granular proliferations on the conjunctiva. The ocular exudate may go from serous to mucopurulent to purulent. Either one or both eyes may be involved. On occasion, a thin film of fibrous exudate develops on the lids and, when removed, reveals a granular,

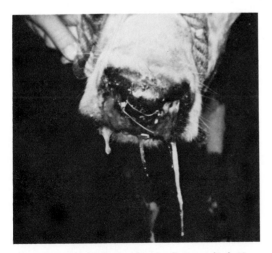

Fig. 4–3. Muzzle of cow showing lesions of infectious bovine rhinotracheitis.

reddened conjunctiva. In some outbreaks, inflammation with clouding of the cornea may develop.

Corneal involvement appears to be an extension of the conjunctivitis, a fact that helps to distinguish this form from pinkeye (infectious bovine keratitis), a condition beginning with ulceration of the center of the cornea. Eye lesions in observed outbreaks are usually healing at the end of the clinical outbreak. Remember that, in rednose, not only a conjunctivitis but also a keratitis may occur, although the keratitis is usually secondary to the conjunctivitis.

In heifers, another form of the disease is characterized by pustular vulvovaginitis. Clinically, there are circumscribed areas of inflammation, with the development of pustules, a fibrinous pseudomembrane, and a yellowish exudate visible on the vaginal floor or the vulvar tuft.

In steers, the virus may produce dermatitis in the anal, perineal, and tail-head regions and exudative lesions on the penis and prepuce.

Confirmed outbreaks of infectious bovine rhinotracheitis abortion have occurred. The virus was isolated from the placenta and from liver, spleen, kidneys, lungs, heart, blood, and pleural fluid of aborted fetuses.

In one such outbreak, none of the animals had been previously vaccinated. An infectious bovine rhinotracheitis respiratory and conjunctivitis outbreak had occurred a few months previously in other cattle on this farm and was evidently the viral source in the outbreak. The abortions occurred at about 6 months of pregnancy, and the only common lesion noted was a perirenal hemorrhage in the fetus. The infectious bovine rhinotracheitis virus has been isolated from fetuses aborted as a result of vaccination, but this is not routinely produced by either the intramuscular or intranasal routes of inoculation.

Experimentally, abortions can be produced at any stage of pregnancy and ordinarily occur 3 to 5 weeks after infection. Some confirmed actual field abortions have occurred before any antibodies were detectable in the dams. Although the clinical entities induced by infectious bovine rhinotracheitis are economically important, the abortion syndrome appears to be increasingly significant as more is learned about the genital form of the disease.

In addition to abortion, there is a marked drop in milk production when lactating cows are infected. In some outbreaks, diarrhea is an important and common clinical finding.

Although encephalitic infectious bovine rhinotracheitis does not appear to be common, it does occur. In Australia, in 1962, the virus was isolated from the brains of cattle showing encephalitis.

DIAGNOSIS

History and signs helpful in differentiating this disease from shipping fever or parainfluenza 3 are as follows:

1. Infectious bovine rhinotracheitis may occur independently of stress, movement, or transportation.

2. A severe conjunctivitis with purulent exudate is indicative of infection with the disease.

3. Unless secondarily complicated, there is no pneumonia; the uncomplicated form involves only the upper respiratory tract.

4. Diarrhea, although observed, is not a common clinical finding, whereas it is often associated with the shipping-fever syndrome.

5. All ages of cattle are affected by IBR, whereas shipping fever and parainfluenza 3 are more common in cattle under 1 year of age.

6. Clinically, the nasal and oral mucous membranes are markedly reddened in infectious bovine rhinotracheitis.

The virus may be isolated from lacrimal, nasal, and vulvar secretions. In instances of abortion, the virus can usually be recovered from the fetus. Identification of the virus can be made by reciprocal cross-neutralization studies or serologic tissue-culture inhibition studies. The disease can be readily reproduced in susceptible calves.

POSTMORTEM SIGNS

Postmortem lesions of rednose are of acute respiratory infection, with marked reddening of the oral, nasal, and tracheal mucosa. Hemorrhagic or purulent exudate with frothing is noted in the nose and trachea and, occasionally, in the large bronchi. Obstruction of the respiratory tract with edema and exudate often causes death by suffocation.

Many small hemorrhages are noted in the upper respiratory mucosa. Mucosal edema is common; regional lymph nodes are enlarged.

PREVENTION

The virus of infectious bovine rhinotracheitis is so widespread that seronegative herds are almost impossible to find. Therefore, isolation to prevent infection is impractical. To avoid clinical disease, one must rely on development of immunity through natural exposure or by vaccination. Because of the possibility of clinical disease from natural exposure, many cattlemen prefer to initiate vaccination programs. There are inactivated vaccines, modified live vaccines, and intranasal vaccines. All serve the purpose of preventing clinical disease. The inactivated and modified live vaccines should be used after the animal is 4 months of age. The intranasal vaccine can be used earlier if necessary. All types can be used on adults, but only the inactivated or intranasal should be used on pregnant animals because there have been reports of abortions caused by some modified live vaccines.

TREATMENT

Treatment with antibiotics for severely affected animals is helpful in suppressing secondary infection but has no effect on the virus.

Shipping Fever

Shipping fever is an acute or subacute infectious disease of cattle, sheep, swine, and rabbits that is characterized by several different syndromes, including acute septicemia and pneumonia, and following shipment or stress. The cause is believed to be a poorly understood complex of viral and bacterial agents. However, Pasteurella multocida and P. haemolytica have been most often isolated from animals in the febrile stage of the disease.

Shipping fever was first described in Germany. In 1880, it was described in the United States and P. multocida was incriminated as the causative organism. In 1912, a bacterin was produced that was partially successful against the disease. In 1917, scientists at the U.S. Department of Agriculture first used the term "shipping fever" and divided the disease into three types. Today, there is still confusion about the exact cause of the syndrome.

Geographically, the disease is encountered throughout the world and frequently causes great economic losses. In the southern United States, the acute septicemic form of the disease is most prevalent, whereas in northern states, the respiratory form is most often encountered. The disease occurs frequently in feeder cattle and sheep, especially when subjected to the stress of shipment. Therefore, shipping fever is most common in areas of heaviest animal production.

CAUSE

The cause of shipping fever is fundamentally difficult to elucidate because the disease has multiple causes. The pattern of the disease suggests that the causative agents are divided into three main categories—stress, viral infection, and bacterial infection. Within each of these categories the various elements appear to be nonspecific, so that the typical shipping-fever syndrome might be the result of any combination of the factors listed. The signs of the disease are not usually acute when only stress and a viral agent are present; however, when a bacterial agent is also present, the signs include pronounced involvement of the respiratory tract.

The bacterium, P. multocida, a non-spore-forming, gram-negative rod, is often considered to be the precipitating cause of the disease, but the signs are seen only in cattle and sheep subjected to stress. The disease results when bacteria invade the respiratory tract of animals with lowered resistance because of stress and predisposing viral infection.

Although the parainfluenza 3 virus is commonly involved, many other viruses have been isolated from cattle with shipping fever. These include infectious bovine rhinotracheitis (IBR) virus, adenoviruses, reoviruses, bovine virus diarrhea (BVD), other herpes viruses, bovine respiratory syncytial (BRS) virus, bovine rhinovirus, influenza virus, and enteroviruses.

The stress factors associated with shipping fever cover a wide range of environmental agents. Cold, stormy weather often triggers the syndrome, but the disease has also been seen during hot weather, especially if associated with such contributing causes as prolonged transit, castration, dehorning, weaning, vaccination, or sudden change of diet. Purely physical forms of stress may lead to an outbreak of the disease on a farm or ranch where the livestock have not been shipped or driven long distances.

TRANSMISSION

Research into the causes of shipping fever has revealed that microorganisms associated with the disease can be found in the respiratory tract of normal animals. Therefore, transmission is most likely to be by contact and by consumption of contaminated feed and water. When animals are coughing, droplet transmission of the infection is significant. Very young calves have a measure of resistance to shipping fever, but tend to lose that resistance at about 4 months of age. Calves may become infected at an early age from the teats of cows but may not show signs until much later.

Shipping fever may be seen in several species, but whether it is transmitted from one species to another is not known.

Shipping fever may occur in all seasons of the year, but most occurrences are seen in the fall, the time of greatest movement of feeder cattle and lambs. Crowded feeder cattle routes become heavily contaminated. Such conditions, plus the stress of shipping, provide increasing exposure of all animals to infection. Stockyards, sale barns, trucks, railroad cars, and feed yards become so heavily contaminated that healthy or recovered animals may become carriers and disseminate the disease widely.

FACTORS INFLUENCING SUSCEPTIBILITY

The increase in the incidence of shipping fever has been attributed to the younger age at which feeder animals are shipped. Calves and lambs weaned just before being shipped are more susceptible because they are excitable, experience a drastic change in feed, and have less resistance to infection in general than do older animals.

Predisposing factors are of a major importance in susceptibility to shipping fever. Much work has been done in tracing the progress of the disease from time of diagnosis backward 2 or 3 weeks to discover the environmental or physiological conditions that had been present. Throughout these studies, certain factors reappeared a number of times and have been termed the *predisposing factors* of shipping fever. The following are the most prevalent:

1. Physiologic and emotional changes

to which cattle and other animals are subjected during shipping.

2. Excitement, exhaustion, and change in feed and water.

3. Irritation of mucous membranes by dust.

4. Overcrowding and long periods of feed and water deficiency.

5. Adverse changes in weather conditions, such as those occurring in autumn or spring.

6. Confinement in drafty or humid and poorly ventilated barns.

7. Malnutrition (mainly vitamin A deficiency because vitamin A helps to maintain healthy mucous membranes).

8. Shipment of recently weaned calves and lambs.

9. Stress—a specific syndrome occurring in the body as a result of hormonal influence in response to nonspecific factors.

The virulence of the organism is increased when transmitted from one animal to another animal. There is always the danger that an animal added to a clean herd may be a carrier and may readily transmit the disease. No role has been found for parasites as a predisposing factor in this disease. Age and sex have little effect on susceptibility.

There is much evidence that shipping fever is a complex disease caused jointly by a virus, bacteria, and environmental stress.

SIGNS

Shipping fever is primarily a respiratory disease, varying from a mild form to rapidly fatal pneumonia. The peracute type has an incubation period of 2 to 5 days, during which the animal is depressed, stands apart from the others, and eats or drinks little. The muzzle appears dry, and the hair coat begins to look rough. The temperature rises to 104 to 108° F, and the pulse becomes rapid. As the disease progresses, the affected animal develops a discharge from the eyes and nose and has difficulty breathing. The ears droop, the animal becomes prostrate, and death may occur in 12 to 24 hours.

The acute type shows more pronounced pulmonary involvement, with thick, copious nasal exudate, rapid breathing, hemorrhage from the nose, soft cough, and respiratory rales. The fever is high; the animal does not eat and rapidly loses weight. At times, hemorrhagic diarrhea develops and the animal dehydrates rapidly. There may also be nervous involvement, evidenced by erratic movements.

In the chronic type, the animal has recovered from shipping fever, sometimes without treatment, but has lost weight and has areas of lung consolidation and abscesses. Such calves may survive but are unthrifty. The mortality rate of chronic cases is variable, but most animals do not live more than a few months following an acute course of the disease.

The signs of shipping fever may vary from feedlot to feedlot and from animal to animal. In some feedlots, signs of the disease may be evident upon arrival of a shipment, whereas in others, the respiratory signs may not appear for several days. Usually, signs appear within the first 2 weeks, but the rate at which signs appear in the animals varies, as do the morbidity and mortality rates. The morbidity usually does not exceed 20% at any one time, and with prompt and adequate treatment, the mortality seldom exceeds 5% of affected animals.

POSTMORTEM SIGNS

The pathogenic agents of shipping fever affect the entire respiratory system. With the first rise in temperature, a mucous nasal discharge develops and fills all the paranasal sinuses. A few hemorrhages and some edema may be found in the mucosa of the larynx and upper part of the trachea. Death results from extensive bronchial involvement, pneumonia, and septicemia.

The pathogenic agents localize in the upper respiratory tract and, because of the lowered resistance caused by stress, are able to invade the mucosa. This invasion leads to generalized septicemia. At necropsy, the most prominent observation is pneumonia. However, there is inflammation throughout the nose, sinuses, larynx, and trachea. The lungs are distended with fluid or fibrin, and the chest cavity contains an excess of straw-colored fluid. There may also be evidence of blood in the stomach and intestines.

DIAGNOSIS

The diagnosis in the field is mainly based on a history of predisposing factors, clinical signs, and, if necessary, postmortem signs. Laboratory diagnosis may not be positive, but the demonstration of Pasteurella organisms in the blood or spleen is presumptive of shipping fever.

Typical signs of pneumonia, fever, loss of weight, nasal discharge, and loss of appetite in cattle about 10 days following a stressing experience are the basis for a diagnosis of shipping fever.

Shipping fever in cattle closely resembles contagious bovine pleuropneumonia, both clinically and at postmortem examination; however, the pleuropneumonia spreads through a susceptible population with greater rapidity. Shipping fever is generally most often observed in cattle following shipment over long distances or in newly weaned calves. The clinical signs and severity of the disease may vary from death in 3 to 5 days to recovery without treatment. The diagnosis is complicated because of the number of diseases that can be confused with shipping fever.

Acute dyspnea is characteristic of fog fever and anaphylaxis, but the onset is usually more sudden, the dyspnea more severe, and the lungs more diffusely affected in shipping fever. Chronic shipping fever may resemble chronic emphysema and lungworm infestation.

The diagnosis of shipping fever in swine and sheep is similar to that in cattle. In swine, shipping fever may be confused with and similar to acute enteric salmonellosis, but the latter, although accompanied by pulmonary involvement, is usually distinguished by signs of septicemia and enteritis.

PREVENTION

The complex cause of shipping fever makes its prevention difficult. Elimination of all the sources of stress would require complete control of the environment and marketing practices. The effect of stress factors can be minimized by preparing cattle for shipment. The preconditioning program for calves destined for the feedlots consists of weaning, castrating, vaccinating, and acclimating to a grain ration well in advance of shipping. The stress of shipping may be minimized by avoiding excessive delay en route and giving animals a clean, dry, uncrowded environment on arrival. Hay and ample clean water, rather than full feed, should be offered.

Control of exposure to infectious agents when moving animals and changing environments is complicated by the large number of etiologic agents. The bacterium, P. multocida, is probably the most important organism to control. Chlamydia and mycoplasma have been involved in bovine respiratory disease, but not consistently. Pasteurella is an opportunist that is potentially available for infection and builds in virulence as more and more animals become infected. Immunization against this organism prior to stress is a reasonable and sometimes effective control and prevention measure. Control of the many viruses is more difficult because of their widespread distribution and presence. It does seem reasonable to attempt to immunize for the most common viruses in relation to the circumstances and age of the animal. It also seems reasonable to attempt to minimize exposure to these infectious agents when moving or changing the environment of groups of animals. Contamination in trucks or vehicles from a previous shipment of animals can be removed to avoid exposing a new group. Preventing animals from passing through previously occupied sale yards or barns can prevent exposure. Avoiding exposure at the destination by isolation for a few weeks is also a practical means to prevent transmission between groups.

Vaccines are available for P. multocida, IBR, BVD, and PI_3, and others are being developed. Vaccination should be accomplished in advance of shipping or stressing. To avoid the problem of immunosuppression by colostral antibodies, modified live virus intranasal vaccines or multiple vaccinations should be used.

TREATMENT

Although overall morbidity percentages may be 20%, some herds experience a much higher percentage. Cattlemen have found that adding sulfonamides or antibiotics to drinking water or incorporating antibiotics in feed helps to prevent severe signs of the disease. The additives must be palatable and must not discourage water or feed consumption. It is practical to "mass medicate" sick animals through feed or water, if they are eating and drinking. The additional stress of moving and handling sick animals should be avoided if the diagnosis and therapy can be accomplished without doing so.

Individual acutely sick animals should be separated from the group and placed in a comfortable area where they can be treated. Antibiotics or sulfonamides must be administered to combat the bacterial infection. For those not taking in nourishment, forced feeding may be necessary. Reports of investigations of effective drugs indicate both success and failure with all drugs in common usage. The best recommendation seems to be to use whatever drug has produced the best results in a particular area.

Recommended Practices for the Control of Bovine Respiratory Disease in the Cow-calf Herd*

BACKGROUND

This management guideline is a joint effort between the National Cattlemen's Association (NCA) and the American Association of Bovine Practitioners (AABP). Cattlemen and veterinarians must continually contend with shipping fever and the respiratory disease complex. It is good economic practice for their management systems to rely on the most effective and proven disease-prevention techniques.

The NCA and AABP formed a technical working group on herd health and bovine respiratory disease to establish good management practices for the industry. The group plans to revise and expand this management guide as needed in the future.

INTRODUCTION

This management outline attempts to present the ideal immunization program. There are regional and area differences in disease incidence and the general health of cow herds.

Your management needs may vary. You may need more or less treatments. *Consult with your veterinarian before changing your current program at all times. Follow the label directions on any product used.*

GENERAL

Respiratory diseases continue to be the major cause of disease loss in beef cattle. The costs to cattlemen for treatment, weight loss, death loss, and culling in weaned calves are estimated to be about a third of a billion dollars annually.

*Reprinted in its entirety with permission of the National Cattlemen's Association and the American Association of Bovine Practitioners.

Approximately 80% of U.S. feeder cattle originate in herds of 50 cows or less. Because of the closed-herd status and the scale of operation, it is sometimes difficult for these producers to appreciate the care and processing these calves should receive to be properly immunized. In addition, the concept of "preconditioning" has been poorly interpreted or badly abused by producer, buyer, and veterinarian alike. Furthermore, some feeders want to buy replacement cattle at the cheapest price and in as thin a condition as possible. They frequently overlook the immediate health status and prior immunization of animals they are purchasing, hoping to compensate for losses that might occur through compensatory gains. Success rates vary considerably.

Preconditioning is the preparation of the calf to better withstand the stress of movement from its production site into and through marketing channels. If a preconditioning program is followed, sickness and death rate will be reduced and weight gains improved. Preconditioning involves adequate castration and dehorning, proper immunization against costly diseases, control of parasites, weaning, and water trough and feed bunk adjustment at the calf's production site.

Preconditioning is a complete health management program. "Pre" means before some event. "Condition" means to process, to prepare. Preconditioning feeder calves means "to prepare them so they can best withstand the stress and adjustment they undergo when they leave their point of origin en route to the feedlot."

In simple terms, preconditioning is a management tool—it is an insurance program—which involves the use of best-known practices to produce and market healthy feeder calves. Basically, preconditioning is common sense and sound husbandry.

"HIDDEN" ECONOMIC LOSSES

Often cattlemen fail to recognize all costs associated with sick cattle. The average sick animal will shrink 10 to 20%. Considerable additional labor is required per sick animal. Medicine, treatment regimens, and death losses are expensive. One study revealed an average 3-day medication cost for a 400-lb. calf is $7.08. A 5% death loss increases the cost of each calf $10 to $20, or 5 to 8%. One time through a chute is considered equivalent to a 7-day feeding period; therefore, it is cheaper to prevent disease than to treat it.

BOVINE RESPIRATORY DISEASE (BRD)

Bovine respiratory disease is difficult to control, highly complex, and not completely understood. BRD usually involves more than one respiratory disease organism; therefore, the role of a single disease organism in the respiratory disease complex is difficult to assess.

DISEASE COMPLEX AND STRESS

Many facets of BRD are influenced by geography, season, transportation, herd management, marketing system, nutrition, vaccination, and the management attitudes of the cow/calf producer and the feeder. Numerous studies have shown that BRD results from the combination of stress plus viral, bacterial, and other infectious agents.

STRESS FACTORS

Stress factors include fatigue, hunger, thirst, dust, anxiety, ammonia buildup, adverse weather, weaning, castration, dehorning, shipping, mixing with other cattle, and unnecessary and/or abusive handling.

BACTERIAL ORGANISMS (PATHOGENS)

Bacterial organisms that have been implicated in BRD are pasteurella, pseudomonas, haemophilus, and other bacteria. Pasteurella multocida and Pasteurella haemolytica are the bacterial organisms most frequently isolated from lung lesions of cattle dying from BRD. Haemophilus somnus appears to be a significant cause of respiratory disease. Other pathogens may be added to this list upon further study.

VIRAL ORGANISMS (PATHOGENS)

Viral organisms that have been shown to be involved in BRD are infectious bovine rhinotracheitis (IBR), parainfluenza 3 (PI3), bovine virus diarrhea (BVD), reoviruses, syncytial virus, rhinoviruses, adenoviruses, and as yet unclassified herpes viruses.

OTHER ORGANISMS

Other microorganisms involved in BRD are chlamydia, mycoplasma, and richettsia. Their role in BRD is not fully understood.

ROUTES OF INFECTION FOR BRD

Bovine respiratory disease is seldom the result of a single factor. BRD usually is caused by a combination of stress, virus infection, and invasion of the lungs by pathogenic bacteria, such as Pasteurella and Hemophilus. Stress undermines the natural defenses built in the lining of the trachea and bronchi; respiratory viruses (such as IBR, PI3, BVD, etc.) further damage these natural defenses. Ultimately, pathogenic bacteria find a wide-open road into the lungs where they localize, multiply, and cause the severe damage we call BRD, or pneumonia, or shipping fever.

VACCINATION TO PROTECT AGAINST RESPIRATORY DISEASE

NOTE: Follow the label directions on any products used.

Viral infections. Immunity against IBR, BVD, and PI3 can be achieved by the administration of virus vaccines to cattle. Modified live and inactivated virus vaccines are available in single or combination forms. The routes of administration of these vaccines are intramuscular (IBR, PI3, BVD) or intranasal (IBR and PI3 only). Both intramuscular and intranasal vaccines provide adequate immunity.

Bacterial infections. Bacterial infections can be controlled with bacterins (vaccines) which are composed of killed organisms. Two injections fourteen or more days apart are needed for adequate protection whenever bacterins are used.

Other organisms. Currently, there are no available immunizing agents for chlamydia, mycoplasma, and rickettsia associated with BRD.

RECOMMENDED IMMUNIZATION AND MANAGEMENT PROGRAMS FOR A BEEF COW-CALF HERD

Calves

Because of differences in climate, geography, production systems, and individual management, it is not possible to make a single recommendation for all areas. Several different management options are presented for each individual cattleman's consideration.

Program "A"
For Young Calves (1-3 months of age)

1. Respiratory diseases
   a. IBR-PI3 (use killed vaccine intramuscularly or modified live vaccine intranasally)
   b. Pasteurella
   c. Haemophilus somnus
2. Other diseases
   a. Leptospirosis (single or multiple strains available)
   b. Clostridial diseases (includes Clostridium chauvoei, C. septicum, C. novyi, C. sordellii, C. perfringens C and D, and C. haemolyticum)
3. Other procedures which should be done at this time:
   a. Implant with approved growth stimulants (except animals to be kept for breeding)
   b. Castrate and dehorn
   c. External and internal parasite control. (Some products are not recommended to be used in very young calves.)

Program "B"
For Older Calves (3-4 weeks prior to weaning)

1. Respiratory disease
   a. IBR-PI3: If killed vaccine was administered at 1 to 3 months of age, it should be readministered as a booster, or a modified live vaccine intranasally or intramuscularly may be used instead of the killed product. However, if this is the initial vaccination and not a booster, use the modified live vaccine intranasally or intramuscularly.
   b. BVD: BVD vaccine is available singly or in combination with modified live IBR virus, and/or PI3 virus, and/or Pasteurella. Since calves are not apt to be heavily stressed when vaccinated 3 to 4 weeks *before* weaning, a "combination" BVD vaccine could be used at this time.

Some cattlemen and veterinarians prefer not to administer BVD simultaneously with IBR-PI3 modified live vaccine intramuscularly because of the added stress on the animal. This is true in very young or heavily stressed animals which can be vaccinated against

BVD 2 to 3 weeks later; in this case, at weaning time, it must be emphasized that calves stressed in any form (e.g., castrated, dehorned, branded, shipped, etc.) should not be vaccinated against BVD; otherwise, adverse reactions could occur.

   c. Pasteurella and Haemophilus somnus: Two injections, 2 to 4 weeks apart, are needed whenever Pasteurella and Haemophilus bacterins are used. If the first injection is given at this time, follow with the booster injection at weaning time.

2. Other diseases (not generally part of BRD complex) which may be considered at this time:
   a. Clostridial diseases booster
   b. Leptospirosis
   c. Vibriosis (heifer and bull calves kept for breeding)
   d. Brucellosis (for heifer calves): Requirements vary among different states. Consult with your veterinarian regarding specific regulations in your state. It is a one-time vaccination and generally must be administered by a licensed veterinarian, or other designated animal health official. All brucellosis vaccinations must be officially reported to the appropriate state agency.

3. Other procedures
   a. Vitamin A (injectable preferred)
   b. Implant with approved growth stimulants (except animals to be kept for breeding)
   NOTE: If your immunization program is begun early enough, both initial and booster shots may be administered prior to weaning. This will reduce stress at weaning and reduce shrink and amount of time required to regain weaning weight. This regime is subject to local practices, individual herd health needs, and various combinations of vaccines. The above recommendations, early immunization, processing of cattle, and other management practices are designated to reduce stress at weaning.
   c. Treat for internal and external parasites.

Calves—Weaning Time

1. If original and booster shots have both been given, no additional immunization is needed at this time. Treat for internal and external parasites, if not done 3 to 4 weeks prior to weaning.

2. If the first vaccination series as listed in Program "A" (young calves, 1 to 3 months of age), above, has been given, give boosters as listed under Program "B" (3 to 4 weeks prior to weaning) and treat for internal and external parasites.

3. For calves that have not previously been vaccinated, several alternatives are feasible, depending upon type of confinement, feed, equipment, availability of labor, and final disposition or destination of the calves. Calves must be handled twice for optimum results; two programs ("C" and "D") are outlined for your selection.

Program "C"
At Weaning

1. Respiratory disease
   a. IBR-PI3 intranasally or intramuscularly (killed vaccine)
   b. Pasteurella bacterin
   c. Haemophilus bacterin
2. Other diseases
   a. Clostridial bacterin
3. Other procedures
   a. Internal parasites
   b. Implant
   c. Vitamin A

14-21 Days Later

(Providing calves are consuming 2 to 3% of body weight of feed, or are on pasture and eating well)
1. Respiratory disease
   a. IBR-PI3 booster if killed vaccine was used at weaning
   b. BVD vaccine
   c. Pasteurella booster
   d. Haemophilus booster
2. Other diseases (not generally considered part of BRD) which may be prevented at this time
   a. Clostridial booster
   b. Leptospirosis bacterin
   c. Vibriosis bacterin
   d. Brucellosis (heifers)
3. Other procedures
   a. Treat for external parasites

Program "D"
At Weaning

1. Respiratory disease
   a. Pasteurella bacterin
   b. Haemophilus bacterin
   c. BVD vaccine
2. Other diseases
   a. Clostridial bacterin
3. Other procedures
   a. Treat for internal parasites
   b. Implant
   c. Vitamin A

14-21 Days Later

(Providing calves are consuming 2 to 3% of body weight of feed, or are on pasture and eating well)
1. Respiratory disease
   a. IBR-PI3 intranasally or intramuscularly
   b. Pasteurella booster
   c. Haemophilus booster
2. Other diseases (not generally associated with BRD) which may be considered at this time
   a. Clostridial booster
   b. Leptospirosis bacterin
   c. Vibrio vaccine (heifers and bulls)
   d. Brucellosis (heifers)
3. Other procedures
   a. Treat for external parasites

ADDITIONAL MANAGEMENT TIPS

High levels of antibiotics may be fed during the weaning period on the advice of your veterinarian. Do not attempt to feed antibiotics unless calves are consuming 2 to 3 percent of body weight of feed. The need and the level of antibiotics should be determined by your veterinarian. Prior to working cattle, consult with your veterinarian concerning the use of epinephrine to treat shock or sensitivity reactions in cattle. It is a potent drug. You should know the clinical signs of shock and sensitivity, indications for epinephrine, and its dosage. Always take time out to observe cattle that have been treated.

Management of Calves at Weaning

1. Calves should be eating some dry feed 2 to 4 weeks prior to weaning.
2. Vaccination procedures should be reviewed and changed as necessary, depending upon health conditions of specific lots of cattle, environmental conditions, and prevalence of various diseases in the immediate area.
3. An adequate fresh water supply is essential, preferably from a source which cattle can see or hear running.
4. Vitamin A prior to or at weaning is generally recommended.
5. Check feed and water consumption—both should increase during the weaning period.
6. Provide good high-quality hay. Calves should be consuming 2 to 3% of body weight of feed before either the feed or water is medicated.
7. Check calves 2 or 3 times daily.
8. Seek professional help from your veterinarian when needed and before a major problem arises.

Marketing and Transportation

1. Minimize stress factors as follows:
   a. It is crucial to get calves moving through marketing channels quickly.
   b. Avoid crowding and bruising.
   c. Avoid conditions of extreme temperature variations, dust, or wetness.
   d. Feed and water calves before shipping.
2. Other factors to improve health:
   a. Upon arrival at the feedlot, cattle should first be fed hay prior to having access to water. Be sure to have adequate water facilities available. Begin a limited feeding of grain and protein supplement.
   b. Segregate sick animals.
   c. Tractor exhaust stacks must be tall enough for gases to clear trailer well.
   d. Avoid ammonia build-up in trucks, yards, barns, or sheds from excess urine, manure, moisture. Ammonia contributes to respiratory disease.
   e. Start adequate treatment promptly. Identify sick cattle and treat as recommended by your veterinarian.

COW HERD, REPLACEMENT HEIFERS AND BULLS

It must be emphasized that vaccination and adequate handling of calves are part of, but not a substitute for, a total herd health management program. It is essential that an adequate breeding herd vaccination program be implemented if maximum benefits are expected from vaccinating and/or preconditioning calves.

The following recommendations are intended to insure immunization of the breeding herd against diseases of recognized significance.

Replacement Heifers and Bulls (generally 10–15 months of age)

The immunization outlined below should be boostered annually, no later than 30 days prior to breeding.
1. Replacement cattle with unknown history status—heifers not pregnant
   a. First working
      1. Immunization: (a) IBR-PI3, (b) Vibriosis, (c) Leptospirosis, (d), Clostridial diseases, (e) Haemophilus, (f) Pasteurella ·

    2. Other treatment: (a) Treat for internal parasites, (b) Vitamin A
  b. Second working (14 to 30 days later)
      1. Immunization: (a) BVD, (b) Leptospirosis booster, (c) Vibriosis booster, (d) Clostridial booster, (e) Haemophilus booster, (f) Pasteurella booster
      2. Other treatments: (a) Treat for external parasites, depending upon grub development and season. (b) If heifers are of eligible age, vaccinate for brucellosis. If heifers are older than of eligible vaccination age, they should be tested, possibly twice, for brucellosis.
2. Replacement cattle sufficiently immunized by calfhood and weaning programs
    This is recommended as optimum management, starting after calves are weaned and assuming they have had at least the minimal recommendations suggested for calves.
  a. Booster vaccinations: (1) IBR, (2) BVD, (3) Leptospirosis, (4) Vibriosis, (5) Clostridial
  b. Other treatments: (1) Internal and external parasites, (2) Vitamin A

Mature Cows and Bulls

Assuming that the breeding herd of mature cows and bulls has been previously immunized, either as calves or as herd replacements, the following booster immunizations are recommended:

Booster immunizations	Not less than 30 days prior to breeding		Last trimester of pregnancy
IBR	X	or	X—Killed or intranasal vaccine
BVD	X		*?
Clostridial	X	or	X
Leptospirosis	X		
Vibriosis	X		

    Frequently veterinarians recommend that IBR, BVD,* and Clostridial immunizations be administered during the last trimester of pregnancy because it conveys a greater passive immunity to the calf. One should be cautioned, however, that, if IBR is administered during the last trimester of pregnancy, it be a killed product or an intranasal vaccine.

    Annual boosters are frequently recommended. However it is important that cattlemen consult with their veterinarian as to the appropriate schedule of immunization for their herd.

Special Notice: Brucellosis Status

Cow-calf producers should pay special attention to brucellosis since the infection still exists in many herds in some states. Further regulations regarding vaccination and testing are due to change. If new cattle are to be brought into a herd, they should originate from a negative herd, be isolated from other animals in the herd of destination, and be retested before being commingled with the new herd. Vaccination should be used as recommended by your veterinarian. Vaccinate all eligible heifers for brucellosis. Purchase only vaccinated heifers.

---

*BVD vaccines are modified live virus vaccines and ordinarily should not be administered to pregnant animals. However, there are experimental studies and reports of practitioners having administered BVD vaccines during the last trimester of pregnancy to increase passive immunity in the calf without adverse effects. We are cautioned again, however, that all biologic products should be administered in accordance with recommendations of the manufacturer.

TABLE 4-1. A Summary of Practices Recommended for the Control of Respiratory Disease in a Beef Cow-Calf Herd

	Calves' Age	Immunizations Against BRD	Other Immunizations That May Be Considered	Additional Procedures
Program "A"	Young calves: 1–3 months old	IBR/PI3: killed vaccine intramuscularly or intranasal modified live vaccine Pasteurella Haemophilus somnus	Leptospirosis Clostridial diseases: the "7-way" bacterin is preferred	Castrate and dehorn Implant (except animals to be kept for breeding) with approved product
Program "B"	Older calves: 3 or 4 weeks before weaning	IBR/PI3: booster vaccination given at 1-3 months of age (may use killed vaccine, or intranasal vaccine, or live intramuscular vaccine) —Use only modified live vaccine if this is the first vaccination BVD: Do not give to stressed or very young calves. Not always recommended in conjunction with live IBR/PI3 vaccine. Often given at weaning time. Pasteurella and Haemophilus somnus: booster shots if given earlier (1-3 months old) —if given now for the first time, booster is needed 3-4 weeks later	Leptospirosis Clostridial diseases: a booster is recommended at this time Vibriosis: for heifers and bull calves kept for breeding Brucellosis:—only heifers —state regulations vary; consult with your veterinarian	Vitamin A: Injectable vitamin is preferred Implant:—use approved product —do not implant animals to be kept for breeding Parasite control: —internal —external
Program "C"	Weaning time	IBR/PI3:—give intranasal vaccine or —killed vaccine (in muscle) Pasteurella and Haemophilus somnus: give first shot	Clostridial bacterin: the "7-way" is recommended	Parasites: treat for internal parasites Vitamin A: the injectable is preferred Treat for external parasites
	14-21 days after weaning	IBR/PI3: if killed vaccine was given at weaning, a second shot of killed vaccine is needed now. BVD vaccine Pasteurella and Haemophilus: give booster	Clostridial diseases: a booster is needed now Leptospirosis bacterin Vibriosis: for replacements	
Program "D"	At weaning	Pasteurella and Haemophilus: first shot BVD vaccine	Clostridial bacterin: first shot Clostridial diseases: booster Leptospirosis bacterin Vibriosis bacterin Brucellosis: heifers only	Parasites: treat for internal parasites Vitamin A: injectable Parasites: treat for external parasites
	14-21 days after weaning	IBR/PI3: use modified live vaccine, either intranasal or intramuscular Pasteurella and Haemophilus: booster		

At Weaning Time—If initial and booster shots have been administered as outlined in Programs "A" and "B," no additional immunizations are needed at this time.

—If the first vaccination series as listed in Program "A" was given but was not followed by Program "B" (3-4 weeks before weaning), give boosters listed in Program "B" at weaning time.

—If calves have not been vaccinated at all before weaning, Programs "C" and "D" are offered. It must be emphasized that Programs "C" and "D" are not always an adequate substitute for Programs "A" and "B"; there may be a degree of risk when calves receive various

CHAPTER 5
Diseases with Signs of Musculoskeletal Changes

Four species and a variety of diseases causing lameness are represented in this chapter. Lameness may be a manifestation of altered locomotion or of an altered stance while stationary. The alteration is usually the result of pain either from bearing weight or moving body structures. What may appear as lameness may be altered movement of a leg because of pain from an adjacent structure, such as an acutely swollen mammary gland. Although the muscle damage of blackleg and the arthritis of erysipelas cause lameness, both are contagious, infectious diseases that cause a variety of systemic signs as well as lameness.

RECOMMENDED READING

Adams, OR: Lameness in Horses. 3rd Edition. Philadelphia, Lea & Febiger, 1974.

Amstutz, HE: Bovine Medicine and Surgery. 2nd Edition. Chap. 19. Santa Barbara, American Veterinary Publications, 1980.

Dunne, HW, and Leman, AD: Diseases of Swine. 4th Edition. Chap. 30, Sect. 3. Ames, IA, Iowa State University Press, 1975.

Greenough, R: Lameness Diseases of Cattle. Edinburgh, Oliver & Boyd, 1972.

Jensen, R: Diseases of Sheep. Chap. 15. Philadelphia, Lea & Febiger, 1974.

Leman, AD, et al.: Diseases of Swine. 5th Edition. Chap. 43. Ames, IA, Iowa State University Press, 1981.

Cattle Lameness

Cattle become lame for a variety of reasons. Lameness is a sign of pain resulting from movement of parts of a leg or adjacent body structures or from impact and bearing of weight. Most lameness is the result of injury or infection of the feet.

FOOT ROT

The most common disease of the feet of cattle is aptly called "foot rot" because of the odor from the lesion as the disease progresses. The affected area is in the interdigital space, and the disease is more properly termed an "interdigital phlegmon." The area between the claws becomes swollen, red, hot, and painful. The swelling may extend up the pastern to the fetlock. The animal avoids using the affected foot and is obviously lame.

Foot rot occurs in cattle of all ages and in all types of environments. It is most commonly observed in cattle that congregate in damp, overly contaminated areas. However, foot rot is also observed in cattle on dry rocky pastures, on frozen lots, or confined to barns or stables. It is caused by two organisms, Fusobacterium necrophorum and Bacteroides melaninogenicus, which invade the soft skin area between the claws. Infection is helped by breaks in the skin resulting from injury.

The disease may progress with the infection invading deeper tissues and the joints of the digits. The resulting damage may be so severe that it causes permanent disability. The disease may also resolve or heal without treatment; the swelling may subside, lameness may disappear, and the area between the claws may slough as a chunk of dead tissue.

Cattle with infected feet contaminate the soil and provide a source of infection for other cattle. Therefore, one of the control measures is the removal of cattle from areas of contamination and the separation of lame cattle from the herd. Areas around feed bunks and water tanks are often badly contaminated because of the heavy traffic in a concentrated area. Another method of control attempts to reduce the contamination by spreading lime in areas of concentration. Feeding of iodine compounds, either mixed in a grain supplement or in a salt mixture, has been used effectively to prevent the disease. However, recent concern over increasing levels of iodine in meat and milk may result in regulations limiting the allowable intake of iodine by food animals.

Treatment of "foot rot" is sometimes effective through the administration of antibiotics or sulfonamides to cattle with acute early infection. Sometimes the interdigital space needs to be medicated and bandaged to aid healing. Advanced cases may require amputation of the affected claw to avoid permanent lameness. The most common cause for lack of response to treatment is misdiagnosis. All lameness in cattle is too easily lumped under the term "foot rot," and this either delays or causes omission of an examination to determine if there are other causes for lameness that do not respond to "shots." There is no substi-

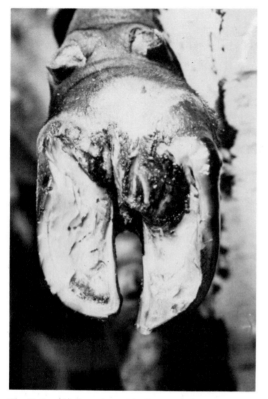

Fig. 5–1. Heel erosion with abscess and undermining of sole.

tute for the disagreeable chore of closely examining the foot to look for nail punctures or other diseases.

HEEL SCALD, STABLE FOOT, OR HEEL EROSION

This disease is also fairly common in cattle. It usually occurs in cattle confined to moist, manure- and urine-contaminated areas. The disease is caused by an organism called Bacteroides nodosus, the same organism as causes sheep foot rot. Although the infection is usually mild, it can progress to serious lameness and disability.

The early signs are slight lameness or reluctance to move. The horn of the heel becomes pitted or dimpled, and the skin above the horn is inflamed. This may progress to erosion of the heel (Fig. 5-1) and extend forward under the sole of the hoof. The erosions and separation of the sole

provide access for further contamination, which may result in an infection migrating to deeper tissues and upward along the tendons. Severe arthritis and bone infection result and are almost impossible to correct. A complication may result from the animal shifting the impact of the claw forward from the painful heel. The concussion of impact, which is normally absorbed by the digital cushion at the heel, is received by the sole, causing a bruise and eventually a sole ulcer (Fig. 5-2).

This condition is prevented by removing animals from the damp contaminated environment. It is also helpful to force the cattle to walk through a 1% formalin foot bath. A stronger solution may be used, but care must be taken to avoid injury to the skin above the hoof.

Treatment is undertaken by cutting away the dead and undermined horn to expose the area to air and by applying formalin or packing with an antibiotic. The outside wall should remain as a bearing surface. As much of the sole as possible should also remain.

SOLE ULCERS

Ulceration of the sole surface of a claw is caused by bruising. Abnormal shifting of impact because of painful heels, excessive wear that thins the horn of the sole, or bruising by rocks and stones to a sole softened by prolonged damp environment may initiate a subsolar bruise. Inspection

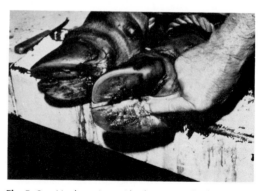

Fig. 5–2. Heel erosion with ulceration of sole.

of the sole shows darkened spots under unpigmented horn. The bruised area may thin, and a raw granulating mass of soft tissue may be exposed. Infection of this lesion is common. Migration of the infection into deeper tissue may cause necrosis of bone, arthritis, and progressive tendonitis.

Sole ulcers may be predisposed by foot and leg conformation. Abnormal weight distribution or a rolled outside wall of the lateral claw seems to make the foot more susceptible to sole ulcers. Excessive trimming weakens or softens the sole, thereby making it more susceptible to bruising.

All the potential causes must be considered in an effort to prevent sole ulcers and infection. Feet should be trimmed to restore a concave sole surface, leaving the wall as a bearing surface and the horn of the sole firm. Cattle should not be subjected to prolonged periods on wet concrete. Such conditions as heel erosion should be recognized and corrected before lameness occurs. Abnormal hoof growth, such as "roll claw," should be corrected as much as possible by periodic trimming.

Treatment of sole ulcers is best accomplished by cleaning and trimming the necrotic area, packing with antibacterial medication, and bandaging. If the opposite claw of the pair is unaffected, it may be extended by fixing a block of wood to it or by forming a plaster-of-paris pad on the sole to give the injured claw relief from any contact with the ground. Thus relieved, the animal spends more time standing and walks without lameness because of relief from pain. Healing of the ulcer is also facilitated without the constant irritation of ground contact.

PUNCTURE WOUNDS

Stepping on sharp objects may cause a deep puncture of the horn of the hoof sole. Nails, wires, wood splinters or thorns, and glass splinters cause puncture wounds. Infection deposited by the puncturing object causes a deep painful abscess, which causes lameness. Swelling from such a wound may not be noticeable, and the wound itself may be difficult to find. Careful cleaning and inspection by scraping the sole with a knife is necessary to find the point of entry. While cleaning or scraping the sole, the offending object may be found buried with the exposed end level with the surface of the sole.

If the object is still in the foot, it must be removed and the wound irrigated or packed with an antiseptic, such as 7% tincture of iodine. If an abscess is found or if drainage of foul fluid indicates an abscess, the horn must be pared away liberally to expose the tract and permit drainage and treatment. Treatment may require packing an iodine-soaked pledget of cotton into the open area or simply swabbing with no packing or bandage. Because cattle are not highly susceptible to tetanus, the need for tetanus antitoxin is a matter of judgment.

Other foot diseases include fractures, sprains, dislocations, proliferative growths, and fibromas. These diseases are not common but must be differentiated from other foot diseases that cause lameness.

ARTHRITIS

Arthritis or inflammation of joints is not uncommon in domestic animals. Although any joint may become inflamed, some are more susceptible than others in cattle. If joints become inflamed, the resulting pain from movement is evident as lameness. Abnormal stance or movement to protect or avoid moving the painful joint aids in determining the source of the lameness.

Joints are structured for the smooth movement of surfaces in contact. The surfaces are therefore smoothed by a cartilage covering instead of rough bone. This surface requires lubrication furnished by fluid (synovia) contained in a capsule surrounding the joint. The joint must absorb shock by some yielding of the contact surface. When a joint is moved beyond its normal range, the ligaments holding it together are overstretched or torn, contact surfaces may be damaged, and the joint segments may become dislocated. The natural response to traumatic injury to a joint is swelling, pain, and altered function.

Joints are of several different types depending on the use. There are hinged joints, sliding joints, and ball-and-socket joints. The hip joint is a ball-and-socket type; the leg joints may be hinged, sliding, or a combination of these types.

A dislocation of the hip (coxofemoral) joint is a serious cause of lameness in cattle. The ball part of the joint on the femur pops out of the socket (acetabulum) of the pelvis. This is usually caused by an abnormal positioning of the hind leg resulting from a fall or awkward recumbent attitude (e.g., a cow slipping on ice and falling with the hind legs out to both sides, or a cow struggling to get up from slippery ground and having both legs extended to the rear, or a cow with poor coordination or control resulting from milk fever struggling to rise). This type of injury occurs most frequently in dairy cows because of their relatively awkward mobility and their bulky, heavy rear quarters resulting from the extensive mammary system.

Although the dislocated joint can be repositioned correctly if done immediately after the injury occurs, the shallow characteristic of the acetabulum in cattle, plus the possibility of chipping the bony rim of the socket at the time of injury, makes the prognosis for success poor. Lightweight athletic cattle of the beef breeds may adjust to the dislocation over a period of time and may survive, although lame. While moving or standing, the leg will be rotated either inward or outward depending on the direction of the dislocated parts of the joint. A heavy, awkward dairy cow so affected frequently refuses to stand or cannot stand.

Injuries to the stifle joint may result from overextension of the hind leg. Overextension to this joint may result in rupture of the ligaments holding the femur and tibia in position, thereby resulting in damage to the joint surface. Lameness is shown by lack of attempt to flex the joint while walking or bearing weight. Although the extent of injury may be determined by radiographs, manipulation of the joint may disclose the abnormal movement caused by the rupture of the ligaments.

Stifle-joint injuries are more common in post-legged or very straight-legged animals. Breeding bulls with very straight hind legs may rupture stifle ligaments during the act of natural service. The practice of trimming or examining feet by tying a rear leg that is extended to the rear may predispose the animal to ligament rupture, especially if the animal should fall with the leg still tied.

Repair of stifle injuries is accomplished by stall rest or the use of a restrictive walking cast or splint. Injury to the shoulder and elbow joints is uncommon and is the result of violent trauma to the foreleg.

The joints in the lower leg often become inflamed or infected by a process starting from the feet. Extension of abscesses to the joints between the third, second, and first phalanges causes severe lameness and often permanent damage. Acute foot rot or sole abscesses frequently extend upward to involve the fetlock area. The area up to and including the fetlock may be swollen and painful. The animal often refuses to bear weight on the affected leg.

Treatment of severe arthritis resulting from an infection is directed toward controlling the infection with poultices and drainage. Surgical removal of the claws with severe bone and joint involvement may be necessary.

A natural response to mild joint injury or irritation is an increase in production of joint fluid (synovia) to lubricate the surfaces. This increase may be in response to an injury or sprain or it may be caused by the animal lying on a hard surface that results in contusion of bony leg joints, such as the hock or carpus. This puffy fluid swelling should not be assumed to be an abscess requiring drainage. Indiscriminate nonsterile lancing of this swelling may turn a harmless natural distention of a joint into a fulminating, lethal, systemic infection.

MUSCLE OR NERVE DAMAGE

The lameness resulting from muscle changes caused by the disease, blackleg, is discussed later. Deep bruising of muscle as a result of cattle butting or fighting is not uncommon. Violent trauma from falling or prolonged pressure of recumbency also causes muscle damage.

Several common nerve injuries cause lameness in cattle. Damage to the radial nerve causes an inability to extend the foreleg. The elbow appears dropped, and the animal drags the leg with the front of the foot on the ground. This injury may be caused by the animal lying broadside on a hard surface for several hours, as might occur during a prolonged attempt to deliver a calf while lying on a rocky hard surface. Large heavy cattle may refuse to stand without the use of one foreleg, whereas young lightweight heifers may be able to stand. If the injury is not too severe, there may be recovery with time. Nursing care during recovery is the only possible treatment.

Damage to the obturator nerves, which control the muscles of adduction of the hind legs, is sometimes the result of the delivery of a large calf from a small heifer. The heifer so affected cannot hold its legs together when standing, and when attempting to move, its rear legs splay out to the side. If unable to stand, the typical recumbent attitude is characterized by the rear legs extended out to both sides. This extension could cause hip dislocation, as previously discussed.

Successful recovery from such damage depends on the amount of nerve damage. Nursing in a well-bedded area for a week to 10 days is sufficient to indicate if there is recovery in control of the legs. Tying the hind legs together to prevent dislocation is sometimes necessary.

A form of muscle spasm of the rear legs of calves is known to be hereditary. The

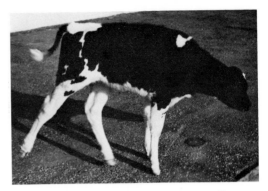

Fig. 5–3. Spastic extension of hindleg of a calf.

disease occurs primarily in calves 2 to 6 months of age. The calf carries one hind leg stiffened straight behind and toward the opposite side and is unable to stand on the leg (Fig. 5-3). The other leg is bearing weight but is held stiff and straight. The muscles above the hock on the rear of the affected leg are hard and taut. The condition is exaggerated with excitement. There is no relief from the condition as the calf grows. The spasm can be corrected by surgically removing segments of the nerve supplying the gastrocnemius muscle. Surgical correction of one leg is usually followed by the occurrence of the same condition in the other rear leg. Although the calf can be restored to normal by surgery, the animal should not be considered for breeding because the condition is heritable.

Another hereditary spastic condition of mature cattle involves both rear legs and is referred to as "crampiness" or "crampy." It occurs in cattle over 3 years of age and is rather mild at first; it becomes progressively more noticeable as years go by. Affected cattle appear normal most of the time and occasionally are seen stretching their rear legs to the rear. Excitement or stimulation of an animal may cause exaggerated stiffening, and muscles of the hind legs feel taut and trembling. Although the episodes are intermittent and most animals can keep up with their herd mates, arthritis develops with time and the animal becomes generally uneconomical. Although considered to be a simple recessive genetic defect, affected animals should not be considered good breeding stock.

Spinal cord injuries are rather common in cattle. Cows riding each other during estrus or large bulls breeding heifers may cause a degree of spinal nerve damage. The affected animal may appear to be weak or incoordinated, may knuckle at the fetlock (Fig. 5-4), and may lose ability to move the tail. Often, these signs are temporary and subside with confinement and rest. However, some animals may be so severely affected that they are unable to stand. When the spinal cord damage is the result of an injury, the onset of signs is sudden. Pressure in the spinal canal from a tumor or abscess causes a gradual loss of

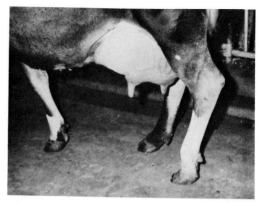

Fig. 5–4.　Knuckling of fetlock due to tibial nerve damage.

leg control over several days or weeks. Tumors of bovine leukosis are credited with causing this type of spinal pressure.

Equine Founder (Laminitis)

Pain in the feet of an animal whose usefulness depends on speed, strength, and mobility is a disaster. Such pain happens frequently to horses, sometimes mildly and sometimes so severely that the animal must be destroyed. Laminitis is inflammation of the junction between the horn of the hoof and the bony skeleton. This junction is formed by interlocking leaves or lamina richly supplied with a network of capillaries and blood vessels. Inflammation results in damage to the circulation of the hoof and excruciating pain. Mild episodes may resolve themselves without noticeable damage. More severe occurrences may result in circulatory changes that alter the rate of growth of the hoof wall, causing so-called "founder rings" or "ski foot" type of appearance. Very acute laminitis may result in complete separation of the lamina with rotation of the tip of the last digit (third phalanx) to penetrate the sole of the hoof.

Cause

The causes of laminitis range from various dietary insults to galloping a horse on a hard-surfaced road. Changes in diet that cause a lactic acidosis have been consistently linked to the occurrence of laminitis. Excessive intake of carbohydrates from overeating grain or a continuous diet of feed high in carbohydrates may often result in laminitis (or grain founder). Rapid intake of cold water by an overheated horse or even eating lush spring pastures may result in laminitis. The stress of an acute infectious process, particularly retained placenta or metritis in a mare, may result in an endotoxemia and subsequent laminitis. The various causes have influenced the use of the terms grain founder, grass founder, post-parturient founder, and road founder.

Signs

The first evidence of acute laminitis is a reluctance to move. Because laminitis occurs more commonly in the front feet, the animal usually attempts to displace weight to the rear by extending the front feet and bringing the rear legs farther forward under the center of the body. There is a characteristic increase in the strength and rate of the digital pulse. There may be an elevation of body temperature and profuse sweating. If all four feet are affected, the weight will be distributed evenly and will cause no change in the stance of the horse. However, a horse affected in all four feet is reluctant to move and lies down if possible. Palpation of affected hooves may disclose an increase in local temperature.

Prevention

Because the causes are management related, they can be controlled and prevented. In addition, when laminitis is suspected as a sequel to retained placenta, severe systemic infection, or acute indigestion, such therapy as mineral oil given orally and electrolytes given intravenously is used to prevent formation and absorption of endotoxins. Horses or ponies that are known to be highly susceptible may require a strict adherence to a high-roughage, low-grain diet.

Treatment

Treatment for acute laminitis should accomplish four objectives: remove or counter the existing causes, relieve pain, restore circulation, and prevent rotation of the coffin bone (third phalanx).

If the cause is dietary, the horse is removed from the source of feed, and mineral oil and detoxicants are administered orally. If the cause is a retained placenta, therapy to expel the placenta and intrauterine medication are administered.

To relieve pain and restore circulation, the digital nerves are blocked with a local anesthetic, and drugs are given to reduce the vasocontraction of the vessels in the hoof. Anti-inflammatory drugs, such as phenylbutazone, may be useful for further relief. Exercise by walking is also prescribed to restore normal circulation to the inflamed area. Once the local anesthesia is effective, the horse is usually willing to walk.

To avoid rotation of the coffin bone and subsequent penetration of the sole of the hoof by its tip, one should encase the foot in plaster of paris to assure pressure on the frog and to shift the burden of the weight from the sole to the hoof walls.

Treatment to include all these measures may have to be continued for many days to assure the animal's return to normal. During this time, the horse should receive a bland diet of well-cured hay and fresh water without grain. Exercise should be limited to controlled walking.

Treatment of chronic deformities resulting from laminitis is directed toward the long-term regrowth of a normally shaped hoof. Such treatment is costly and time consuming and is not always successful.

Blackleg and Malignant Edema

These two diseases are combined in one chapter because their signs are similar, both are caused by similar organisms, and prevention measures are almost always combined.

BLACKLEG

Blackleg is a sporadic, acute, infectious, noncommunicable disease of livestock. It is characterized by gas-filled swellings in the heavy muscles, especially of the hindleg, which crepitate or crackle when palpated. This disease is sporadic in nature and affects mainly young cattle and sheep, although occasionally goats and wild ruminants may be affected. Blackleg is caused by Clostridium chauvoei, one of the gas-producing organisms commonly contaminating pastures and feedlots.

Geographically, blackleg has been found in all parts of the world where cattle are raised and where cattle and sheep are pastured on low-lying, marshy pastures or, more frequently, on well-irrigated pastures.

Historically, blackleg is one of the older diseases known to cattle; however, a positive diagnosis of the condition was not made until 1875. Prior to that time, blackleg had been confused with anthrax, but in 1875, the disease was finally differentiated and the organisms causing the disease were cultured.

Cause

Blackleg is one of the clostridial diseases. It is caused by C. chauvoei, a gas-producing, spore-forming, gram-positive, rod-shaped bacterium. The microorganism occurs singly in cultures, and the spore develops subterminally. In the natural state, the spore form is most often found on contaminated pastures. The vegetative form, however, may be found in the diseased muscles of animals that have died of this disease. The organism growing in the animal body produces a toxin that is not, however, as potent as the toxins produced by other clostridial microorganisms. There are several antigenic strains of the blackleg organism, but there are no differences between the sheep and cattle strains. The spore stage of the microorganism is resistant and remains viable on pastures, contaminated feed, and bedding for a considerable length of time. C. chauvoei exists in the soil and is ingested on the forage from the contaminated pastures. Multiplication of the vegetative stage takes place in the intestinal tract of farm animals; the spores enter the blood where they circulate until a focus is established. At that time, the spore organisms change into the vegetative state and rapidly develop, causing the gross appearance of the disease. The spore-forming organisms are found in most parts of the United States but primarily in areas where low-lying pastures, at times marshy or swampy, predominate.

Transmission

The primary source of infection is usually considered to be ingestion of contaminated spores, which enter the digestive tract with contaminated feed and water. Wound infections, whether from tick bites, scratches, wire cuts, animal bites, or any other traumatic experience (such as castration or docking), provide a means of entry for the organism into the blood. Soil infection is considered to be the primary source because spores of the microorganism are found both outside and inside the body of an infected animal. If the pasture becomes infected, it remains so permanently.

In sheep, wounds of any kind, whether accidental (as from shearing cuts, injury from fences, and similar causes) or intentional (as from docking, castration, or vaccination procedures) should be looked on as potential avenues for the entrance of the disease-producing organisms. Microorganisms commonly enter the body when sheep are dipped for scab, lice, or sheep ticks immediately after shearing. Too often, this operation is careless, resulting in scratches and cuts of the animal's skin. The dip serves as a focus for the collection of microorganisms, which may then enter the body through the lesions described. When this occurs, the results are often disastrous, as treatment is generally ineffective after the disease has developed. The disease may occur in ewes from infection of wounds of the genital tract produced at lambing time. In rams, lesions have appeared about the head from infection of wounds received when butting and fighting. Grass cuts on legs of both sheep and cattle may serve as a means of infection through the skin.

Factors Influencing Susceptibility

Young cattle from 4 months to 2 years of age suffer from blackleg, as do sheep and goats of most ages. However, cattle that have not been vaccinated against the disease or that have not been in an area where the disease is prevalent may succumb at an older age. Wild ruminants (such as deer), swine, and laboratory animals are also infected on occasion. Older cattle are usually resistant to the disease because they have either recovered from an inapparent bout of infection or because they have not had access to an infected area and thus have not experienced the disease-producing organisms. In this way, a measure of resistance may be considered a part of disease prevention. There is no evidence of physiologic immunity to this disease nor is there a relationship between the disease and sex or breed. The disease is most often seen in well-nourished young cattle at about the time of weaning. Most instances appear in the fall, early winter, and spring, but they can occur at any time regardless of weather or feeding conditions. Herd outbreaks commonly occur among unvaccinated beef calves soon after weaning in the fall. Livestock maintained on cultivated land, especially irrigated pastures, or on low, swampy regions are more susceptible to the disease than are cattle or sheep maintained on dry, upland pastures. Cattle presumably contract infection through ingestion of contaminated food, soil, or water rather than from the introduction of the microorganism through wounds or injuries, as occurs with sheep.

Clinical Signs

In cattle, signs usually appear sporadically or spontaneously and are unassociated with wounds or other injuries. Affected animals are usually in good condition, and the disease appears when they are turned out to pasture. The incubation period is from 1 to 5 days (usually less than 3 days), and the course of the disease is rapid, from 24 to 60 hours. There is an acute rise in temperature to 106°F. When signs are seen, the animal appears lame and resents movement. The swellings commonly appear in the hindlegs or hip regions and are hot and painful. Later, the swellings are cold, and the animal does not evidence pain when they are palpated. The animal may be found lying on his side, with legs extended and the swellings filled with gas (Fig. 5–5). There is usually a dry, crackling sound as the result of this gas accumulation under the skin. The skin appears dry and dark over the areas where gas is not-

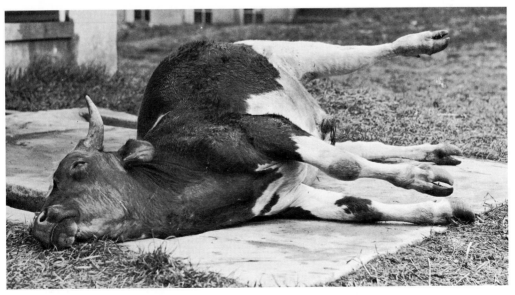

Fig. 5–5. A young steer that has died of blackleg.

ed. Respiration increases rapidly and there is a rapid, thready pulse. Just prior to death, the temperature falls and the animal becomes comatose. In most instances, the first sign of disease is a dead animal.

The signs in sheep are different from those in cattle. In sheep, age is not a factor in incidence of disease. Sheep of all ages may be affected, from lambs a few days old to ancient ewes and rams. A considerable time may elapse between ingestion of the spores and the appearance of signs in sheep. Although spontaneously developed lesions may occur in sheep of all ages, serious outbreaks usually follow such traumatic farm operations as shearing, crutching, dipping, docking, and castration. Because of the slow development of the disease in sheep, they are rarely found dead without premonitory signs. These signs include lameness, reluctance to move, crepitating swellings on various parts of the body, rise in temperature, and inability to stand. Afterward, the animal dies quickly.

Postmortem Signs

Once organisms of blackleg have entered the body from the spore state, they tend to localize within the crypts of the intestines, where they find an anaerobic atmosphere in which to develop. Once they enter the circulation, however, they circulate until they localize in injured or poorly drained muscle tissue. There, the development of necrotic tissue provides a favorable environment for the growth of the vegetative stage of the bacterium. Toxin liberated by the vegetative stage of the microorganism causes local necrosis of the muscles in the area surrounding the foci of infection. The gas produced breaks up the tissue and provides a gaseous, hemorrhagic inflammation, which then is evidenced by crepitation. The toxins liberated cause high temperatures, rapid respiration, degenerative changes, and death.

There is little putrefaction as the result of a gross infection with C. chauvoei organisms. However, large crepitant swell-

ings or changes may occur, although on occasion, such changes may not be extensive. Upon excising the skin, the muscle color is dark, with light streaks and gas pockets that produce a pungent, rancid odor. The fluid exuding from a cut portion of skin is frothy as a result of gas bubbles within the fluid. If blackleg is suspected, it is best not to open the skin. If the skin is removed, it will be hemorrhagic immediately under the surface. In sheep, spontaneously occurring lesions are often small and deeply situated, and they may be easily overlooked on autopsy. Consequently, the condition may be confused with other clostridial diseases. Thus, an accurate diagnosis can be made only by laboratory examination of specimens taken from the sheep at time of autopsy. However, when young cattle die suddenly and exhibit gas-filled lesions or swellings of the muscles (primarily of the hindlegs) without any other signs, blackleg must be suspected.

Treatment and Prevention

Signs of blackleg in young cattle are seldom observed in time to save the animal. However, because the disease is not so spontaneous in sheep, they may be treated successfully with a variety of broad-spectrum antibiotics. In areas where expensive animals are kept for breeding purposes, the use of an antiblackleg serum, which provides temporary protection, may also be used. The veterinarian should be contacted immediately whenever blackleg is suspected.

Because blackleg is a disease both sporadic in nature and enzootic in various parts of the country, immunization must be done yearly on infected premises. Blackleg bacterin is used extensively and is safe and reliable for both cattle and sheep. A single injection confers immunity that lasts for several months. Where heavy infection of premises necessitates early vaccination of calves and lambs—before they are old enough to produce strong, active immunity—a second vaccination must be given at about 6 months of age or at the time of weaning. In sheep, vaccination is used not only as a routine measure in blackleg areas, but also as a preventive at the beginning of an outbreak to check further losses. Furthermore, whenever animals die of blackleg the carcasses should be buried deeply, all known blackleg-contaminated ground should be cultivated, and young animals should be kept out of such areas until they have been effectively immunized.

The bodies of animals that have died are the chief source of soil infection. They harbor the microorganisms in large numbers and liberate them from artificial and natural body openings. For this reason, any dead animal should be promptly burned or buried, and with few exceptions, the sick should be slaughtered and disposed of in the same manner. Disinfect all woodwork or utensils that have come in contact with the infection. The surface of the ground may be made safe by burning it over with a heavy layer of straw. Because of the vitality of the spores of blackleg, pastures may remain infected for years, even when kept free of cattle. In some regions where contamination of the soil is limited, the disease may be avoided by a change of pasture. Possibly, in time, an infected pasture may become free of microorganisms if all animals feeding on it are vaccinated.

MALIGNANT EDEMA

Malignant edema is an acute, usually fatal, infectious disease of cattle, sheep, goats, swine, and man. The disease is caused by Clostridium septicum and is characterized by swellings within the body, usually located around a wound into which pathogens have entered or localized in the tissues. The disease produces marked prostration and is often fatal in 1 to 4 days.

This disease was discovered early by Pasteur and co-workers. They cultured the causative bacteria from the blood of a cow in 1877. Koch later produced the disease in cattle and described the organism in great detail.

Geographically, the organism is worldwide in distribution and is found wherever cattle and sheep are raised. However, the disease is not as prevalent on the American continent as on the European and Asian continents.

Cause

The cause of malignant edema is C. septicum, a short, plump rod that grows actively in penetrating or lacerated wounds; it grows anaerobically and produces gas deep within the muscle tissues. The cause is similar in both man and animals. Closely allied with the causative organism are any number of Clostridium organisms found in the soil.

Transmission

The organism gains entrance to the body through cuts, lacerations, and penetrating wounds caused by castration, docking and shearing, vaccination with unclean needle, abortions and deliveries in contaminated surroundings, broken bones, wire scratches, and the bites of animals. The most susceptible hosts are cattle, sheep, and swine, although horses, mules, dogs, and men are also susceptible. There are no premonitory factors affecting susceptibility, and there is no relationship associated with either sex or age. The disease may occur in all species of animals at any time. Although malignant edema is an infectious disease, it is not considered a contagious disease.

C. septicum, the microorganism causing this disease, exists in all fertile soils and in the intestinal tract of herbivorous animals. Whether it multiplies in the soil or merely exists in the soil as spores after being formed by the vegetating organisms in the intestinal tract of animals is not known. Infection ordinarily occurs through contamination of nonaerated wounds, but many instances of this disease cannot be accounted for in this manner.

Clinical Signs

The period of incubation of malignant edema is from 2 to 5 days after a wound has become contaminated. Sometimes the condition occurs more rapidly, depending on the infecting dose and the extent of the wound. Usually within this time, edema-like swelling occurs, primarily involving the subcutaneous tissues and the skin. The organism spreads rapidly, and the lesions may become emphysematous. Blood-tinged fluid may escape at the point of injury or can be withdrawn by hypodermic aspiration. Lameness, fever, increased pulse rate, congestion of the conjunctiva, and marked toxemia appear almost in the order given. Death may occur in 1 to 4 days after the appearance of the initial lesions. When the disease is prolonged, a profuse, foul-smelling diarrhea may be noted. When a genital infection follows abortion or delivery of a dead fetus, swelling of the labia, necrosis of the vagina, and external edema gravitating to the ventral abdomen may occur. Following castration, signs may develop within a few hours or not until several days following the operation. The signs first appear as swelling with serosanguineous exudate from the incision. Later, the swelling becomes more extensive, extending downward to the ventral area. The affected animal becomes toxic, develops a high temperature, shows signs of dyspnea, and dies.

Postmortem Signs

The malignant edema organism, C. septicum, gains entrance into the body with dirt through penetrating wounds. There it finds suitable foci for growth in the necrotic tissue resulting from the trauma. The toxin produced causes edema and gas production, which further disrupts the muscle tissue. Upon postmortem examination, a massive edema due to straw-colored or brownish fluid in the area of the wound is noted. The muscle tissue appears reddish-black and gas bubbles are evident throughout the area. The gas bubbles tend to be subcutaneous rather than intermuscular, as occurs with blackleg. There is usually edematous fluid in the body cavities and in the pericardial sac. Other signs are generalized hyperemia and cyanosis of the tissue. In the field, the condition is diagnosed primarily through a history of traumatic wounds, plus the typical lesions and signs. However, positive diagnosis can only be made by laboratory isolation of the causative organisms.

Prevention

Prophylaxis depends on sanitation and immunization. Immunization is accomplished by using bacterins composed of a combination of organisms. It has become a common practice to include the organisms of both malignant edema and blackleg in a single bacterin for protection against both diseases. For best results, lambs and calves should be vaccinated at the time of castration and again at about 6 months of age.

Because malignant edema organisms continue to multiply for some time after sporulating in the carcasses of dead animals, all carcasses suspected of this disease should be destroyed immediately either by deep burying or burning. A wise precaution against the disease is strict asepsis during such operations as castration, docking, surgery, inoculation, or injection.

Treatment

Malignant edema lesions are difficult to treat. However, some success has resulted from multiple injections of penicillin directly into the site of the lesion. Post-calving lacerations of the vulva are a common site for infection with C. septicum. If the lesion is treated early (before severe systemic signs appear) the result may be a live animal but a large, slow-healing necrotic area at the site of infection.

Ovine Foot Rot

Foot rot, or infectious ovine pododermatitis, is a chronic, contagious, nonsuppurative disease of the feet of sheep and goats. It is characterized by progressive necrosis of the deep layers of the epidermis, separating the horn from the soft tissues and resulting in lameness.

Historically, foot rot has been recognized and mentioned in the literature of Europe for several hundred years. The disease has been known in America since the arrival of the first sheep, but it was not until 1904 that scientists in the U.S. Department of Agriculture discovered the causative microorganisms.

Geographically, the disease occurs worldwide, but the incidence varies appreciably and is most common in areas where heavy stocking is practiced and where rainfall is abundant.

Cause

The disease is caused by two distinctly different bacteria; it does not exist if only one is present. Both of these organisms are anaerobes, that is, they live and grow only in the absence of air. This fact is important in understanding the prevention and treatment of the disease. Of the two organisms, Bacteroides nodosus, a strict parasite that does not live more than a week away from an infected foot, is the primary cause, but Fusobacterium necrophorum must also be present to produce the disease.

The incubation period for foot rot is 7 to 14 days. Therefore, purchased or borrowed animals should be kept under quarantine for 2 to 3 weeks before they are allowed to mingle with noninfected sheep.

The causative microorganisms live and are carried in the dead tissue trapped in overgrown and neglected feet of sheep and goats. Moist, lowland pastures are conducive to rapid overgrowth of the hoof and to lack of normal hoof wear, and are therefore often associated with the disease. However, the disease cannot exist unless the specific bacteria are present.

One or several feet may be affected. Both claws on the affected foot are usually involved. An injury or wound is usually the point of entry of infection, but by the time the disease is recognized, this wound is seldom apparent.

Transmission

In almost all instances, the disease is introduced into a flock through the purchase or borrowing of infected animals. The disease spreads within a flock as a result of infection picked up on pasture, in wet areas around water tanks and water holes, and in filthy pens contaminated by the feet of infected sheep. The infection does not survive long in the presence of air. Pastures that have been free of sheep for 2 to 3 weeks may be considered clean and safe to use.

Foot rot is potentially economically serious in sheep, especially in the larger flocks. The reason for this is twofold: (1) the tremendous amount of time and labor required to eradicate the disease, and (2) the losses in breeding flock and market lambs during the treatment and eradication period.

Contagious foot rot is a specific disease of sheep and goats and is not acquired from contact or association with other species of farm animals. It is totally different from, and should not be confused with, foot rot in cattle.

Factors Influencing Susceptibility

Sheep and goats of all ages, sexes, and breeds are susceptible. Certain breeds have, at times, been claimed to have natural resistance to the disease, but these claims have not been substantiated by field observation or research.

Signs

The first and most obvious symptom is lameness, commencing with a mild inflammation between the claws. As the infection progresses, it causes a break in the skin of the junction with the horn and spreads rapidly under the horn tissue to the sole.

In the early stages of an outbreak, one or more individuals show an area of tenderness, reddening, and puffiness between the toes and on the heels. The foot may feel warmer than normal. The infected areas of the foot then become grayish, and if the dead tissue is trimmed away, a cheesy, yellowish-gray material with a characteristic foul odor can be found. The infection spreads into cracks and pockets, and the sole and horny hoof become separated from the normal soft-hoof structures. When both front feet are involved, sheep are often seen eating and moving on their knees.

Foot rot has been reported in lambs in as early as the sixth day. Needless to say, such lambs and sheep are unthrifty and subject to malnutrition and disease. Death loss from foot rot is rare, but can occur from complications arising as a result of the initial foot-rot problem.

Foot rot does not usually start in the lambs. It is a ewe-flock problem that subsequently spreads to the lambs.

Diagnosis

Foot rot may be diagnosed by clinical signs, flock history, and environment. The causative microorganisms may be demonstrated, although care must be exercised in the interpretation. Lameness and a foul smell are strongly suggestive of the disease.

If the flock has not had foot rot and there have been no flock additions within the past 10 to 14 days, the lameness is probably not caused by foot rot. If the lameness is due to foot rot, neither the foot nor the joints are swollen because the horny portion of the hoof, and not the soft tissue

above the coronary band, is involved. In typical contagious foot rot, there is not an abundance of moist, oozing, foul-smelling discharge.

All sheep have an interungulate or biflex gland between the toes on each foot. If this gland becomes plugged, infected, injured, or otherwise irritated, it may cause lameness. The ability to squeeze a grayish, cheesy mass of material from this gland should not be regarded as a sign of contagious foot rot; it is perfectly normal.

Prevention and Control

Preventive measures for the control of foot rot are based on good practical animal husbandry. By eliminating those factors that predispose an animal to the disease, exposure can be prevented. Preventive measures should be initiated in the dry season and should include elimination of potential mud holes, inspection and trimming of feet of all animals (including rams), application of an approved foot bath, and proper quarantine for all additions to a flock, including those returned from shows, fairs, and salebarns.

The feet on each sheep on the farm or in the flock must be trimmed thoroughly and completely. All pockets, cracks, and crevices should be trimmed and healthy tissue exposed to the air. Once this is done, any good disinfectant can accomplish the remainder of the task. Do not attempt to spot-check sheep that are lame. Foot rot is a flock problem and must be treated on a flock basis. Every animal must be examined, the feet trimmed, and infected animals removed from the flock.

Because the organisms that cause the disease live only in the absence of air, the first and most vital step in the control and treatment of this disease is regular trimming of the feet. By removing all dead and abnormal tissue, air is permitted to reach all parts of the normal foot, and the infecting organisms, if present, can no longer survive.

There is no self cure or recovery for untreated sheep. Likewise, sheep that have been treated and are cured are not immune to future infection. However, if an affected flock is thoroughly and adequately treated and the infection is eliminated, the disease will not recur unless introduced into the flock by the addition of infected animals.

The complete control and eventual eradication of foot rot in sheep depend on accurate diagnosis, prompt and complete compliance with the recommended procedures, and cooperation among producers, veterinarians, feedlot operators, sellers, and carriers.

Swine Erysipelas

Swine erysipelas is an infectious disease mainly of young swine, but is manifested in various ways in cattle, horses, fish, birds, laboratory animals, and man. The causative organism, Erysipelothrix rhusiopathiae, has been incriminated as the cause of nonsuppurative arthritis in lambs and calves, postdipping lameness in sheep, acute septicemia in turkeys, and erysipeloid in man, as well as in diamond-skin disease, arthritis, and heart disease in swine.

Swine erysipelas does not often result in severe herd losses from death, but the great economic loss comes from the general unthriftiness of animals that have recovered from a mild attack or are suffering from the chronic form of the disease.

Geographically, erysipelas is worldwide in distribution and is considered a serious economic disease wherever swine are raised. In the United States, swine erysipelas has been reported from every part of the country and from most states.

Historically, the microorganism now known to cause swine erysipelas was first isolated from a mouse in Europe in 1878. The disease was first described in swine in 1885 and in man in 1887.

In the United States, the specific organism of swine erysipelas, E. rhusiopathiae, was first isolated in 1921 by scientists at the Bureau of Animal Industry from a tissue injury in a Texas hog. The organism was obtained from a specimen of skin showing a "diamond-skin" lesion. Such lesions, typical of those described in European countries as the result of infection

with swine erysipelas, had been observed in the United States for many years, but the disease was called diamond-skin disease. Swine erysipelas was not considered to be present in this country before the isolation of the organism. After this discovery, other workers isolated the organism from lesions in the joints and other tissues of the bodies of swine. It was then recognized that swine erysipelas definitely existed, apparently in a chronic form, in certain parts of the United States. Although the infection appeared to be confined principally to the corn belt, it may have existed in many other states in a chronic, low-grade form.

Cause

Swine erysipelas can be readily isolated from all tissues of pigs showing signs of the disease and from the tonsils of normal swine.

The causative microorganism, E. rhusiopathiae, is small and rod shaped, either straight or curved. It is gram-positive and may have a beaded appearance when viewed under a microscope. It is nonspore-forming, nonmotile, and may form long filaments that do not branch. It survives for long periods in decaying flesh and in water, and is resistant to such preservative processes as salting, smoking, and pickling. The bacterium is susceptible to caustic soda and the hypochlorites, but is resistant to formaldehyde, phenol, hydrogen peroxide, and alcohol.

The microorganism causing swine erysipelas is considered by many to be a saprophyte and to live and multiply in the soil when conditions are favorable. The bacterium multiplies well in warm alkaline soil containing considerable amounts of humus, but dies rapidly in acid soil.

Transmission

Swine erysipelas is an insidious disease, and the manner in which it spreads is not entirely understood. Most likely, however, the disease requires considerable time to make any appreciable headway when introduced into an uncontaminated area. It has probably existed in a chronic form for many years in certain parts of the United States, gradually increasing in virulence until favorable conditions prevail. At such a time, it is manifested by the acute type of the disease.

Because the bacteria can survive for long periods in certain soils, the recurrence of swine erysipelas can readily be brought about by conditions favorable to the microorganisms. On some farms where infection exists, the disease may recur irregularly over a period of several years; however, it may never appear on other farms where the soil is similarly infected. No satisfactory explanation has been made for these differences. Once an infection has appeared on a farm, however, the potential danger exists that it will reappear in subsequent years.

It is not definitely known whether infection proceeds directly from animal to animal or whether the bacteria excreted by an infected animal must pass some part of their life outside the animal body, or otherwise undergo some change, before they can reproduce the disease in susceptible animals. It is generally agreed that cultures of the bacteria reproduce the disease only occasionally when injected into swine. It is also generally believed that some unknown factor, in addition to the microorganism itself, is necessary to bring about infection. The erysipelas microorganism enters the body primarily through ingestion with contaminated feed and water.

The infective agent may also gain entry through abrasions on the skin and mucous membranes; it has been theorized that it may enter the mucosa through lesions caused by parasites. Insect vectors have also been incriminated in the dissemination of this disease to experimental animals, but the significance to the farmer of this means of transmission is unknown.

During an attack of the disease, the causative agent can be found in the blood, urine, and feces. Thus, the surroundings of the animals soon become heavily contaminated. Animals affected with the chronic form of the disease may also pass it to others.

The swine erysipelas microorganism may be harbored in some parts of the bodies of apparently healthy animals, i.e., the tonsils and parts of the intestinal tract. Possibly this is a result of a previous mild infection and recovery, or the organisms may have been picked up from contaminated soil without resulting infection. Such healthy animals may be dangerous to others or may subsequently develop the disease themselves if their resistance is lowered by stress.

The disease occurs most often during the spring, summer and fall of every year. In this country, sows farrow every month of the year, and thus, there is a continuous supply of new pigs susceptible to infection.

In the instance of arthritis in lambs and calves, the causative agent gains entry into the body through slight wounds and scratches and through the untreated naval at birth. Microorganisms may also gain entry at the time of castration, docking, or dehorning unless care is taken to disinfect all wounds and to control the dust in sheep pens and holding yards.

E. rhusiopathiae is a common contaminant in dipping vats used to rid range sheep and cattle of external parasites. Such vats provide a focus from which the microorganisms gain entry into the animal body through small cuts and abrasions, thereby leading to postdipping lameness. The bacteria localize in the joints and in the laminae of the hoof to produce the lesions causing the lameness.

Factors Influencing Susceptibility

Swine of all ages, from suckling pigs to adult animals, are susceptible to the disease. The causative microorganism also affects a variety of fish, birds, and animals, including man. In some parts of this country, the disease is of economic importance in both sheep and turkeys. The bacterium's infectivity to man is evidenced by the number of incidences reported in veterinarians, butchers, and livestock handlers, for whom it is considered an occupational hazard. The so-called fish handlers' disease is caused by infection with the swine-erysipelas microorganism found on the skin of many salt-water fish.

Although it does not bear spores, the erysipelas microorganism contains a waxy substance that is resistant to adverse conditions. It remains active for a month or longer in a cool, dark place. In smears on glass exposed to direct sunlight, it survives only a few days, but remains alive for many days in water. The microorganism is sensitive to heat, however. At 111° F, it is destroyed in 4 days, at 125° F in 15 minutes, and at 130 to 137° F (far below ordinary cooking temperatures) in several minutes.

Live erysipelas microorganisms have been found in putrid material after 4 months. In the flesh of swine, the bacteria are resistant to destruction and have been found living in a carcass buried for 280 days. The microorganisms are only slowly destroyed by salting and pickling, and they have been found alive after 26 days in strong brine.

Because the disease often appears in a low-grade infection, and because animals affected with the chronic form may, in certain circumstances, pass it to normal hogs, animals with a mild infection should be removed from the herd when discovered.

Stress is a factor in erysipelas. Swine experiments have indicated that both vitamin deficiency and ascariasis favor development of erysipelas and may account for some sporadic cases in winter. The incidence of the disease is lowest during the winter months and highest in the hot summer. Whether high temperature and humidity increase the pathogenesis of the microorganism or decrease the animals' resistance, or whether both are factors, has not been determined.

Although swine of all ages are susceptible to erysipelas, suckling piglets of immune dams are not affected for the first few weeks after birth. It has also been postulated that when the dam is affected with chronic arthritis, the period of passive immunity lasts until the piglets are 3 to 4 months of age. However, young pigs are most susceptible to the disease, and swine over 3 years of age are rarely affected. Older animals acquire immunity following either subclinical or inapparent infection.

Factors with a direct bearing on susceptibility usually include one or more of the following: (1) virulence of the bacteria, (2) natural resistance of the pigs to the infection because of maternal antibodies or subclinical exposure, (3) genetic influences, or (4) stress. Stress as a factor of susceptibility may be related to nutrition, atmospheric conditions, overall sanitation on the property, and the virulence of the bacteria in the natural environment. Because the disease-causing bacteria are present on the tonsils and are excreted from the intestinal tract of normal pigs, swine can be reinfected following weather conditions favorable for reproduction of the microorganisms in the soil. It has been demonstrated that the saprophytic development takes place in the top 4 inches of the soil. Thus, rooting pigs are exposed to great numbers of the infecting microorganisms.

Factors altering the physiologic state of the pig can often be associated with an outbreak of swine erysipelas. Such predisposing causes are fatigue; sudden changes in diet; excessive fattening; exposure to cold, high humidity, or warm temperatures; and overfeeding with succulent, high-energy feed.

In handling diseases of swine, owners should always contact veterinarians; this is particularly important in combating actual or suspected outbreaks of swine erysipelas.

Clinical Signs

The clinical signs of swine erysipelas appear in acute, subacute, and chronic forms, although subclinical, inapparent, or unobserved signs may also occur.

Acute Swine Erysipelas

This condition is characterized by sudden onset, and many swine in the herd may be affected at the same time. Only a few may be visibly sick, whereas others may run high temperatures (105 to 110° F). At the higher temperatures, some pigs shiver as though chilled. Affected hogs lie in their bedding, and although their eyes are clear and they appear alert, they are reluctant to move. If forcibly disturbed, they start moving with considerable activity but protest loudly. Because the tissues of the joints are involved in the disease process, many infected swine are undoubtedly in pain when they walk. They make an effort to keep their feet under them, which makes the backbone appear long and strongly arched. After moving about a bit, they drop down on their bedding again. Where considerable swelling at a joint is noted, there may be exostoses (bony growths) that do not disappear when the disease subsides. Animals thus affected are the so-called knotty-legged hogs, or chronics, which harbor the disease organisms in their joints and may act as spreaders of the infection.

Most animals are reluctant to eat during the early stages of the disease and cease to eat altogether as the condition progresses. Often infected pigs stop eating and regurgitate. The feces become hard and scanty, but later diarrhea may develop. Diarrhea is more common in young animals than in older animals.

Several hogs may die quite suddenly. They may appear well at feeding time one evening and be found dead the next morning. There have been instances in which entire herds have died; this situation is rare at present in this country, although it is not uncommon in unvaccinated herds in erysipelas districts of other countries. As a rule, only a few hogs die, some make a complete recovery, and the rest remain unthrifty chronics. The mortality is rarely over 10%, but in any given outbreak, the morbidity may approach 100%.

In hogs acutely ill with swine erysipelas, shortness of breath caused by pulmonary edema (a waterlogged condition of the lungs) may be noted. At times, swellings about the snout make breathing difficult. Nausea and vomiting are not uncommon. Some 24 to 48 hours after the onset of the disease, irregular red patches, neither tender to the touch nor swollen, may be noted on the lighter parts of the skin. Such areas may remain localized or may enlarge and run together until the greater part of the body surface is involved. Death is sudden and is usually preceded by respiratory distress brought about by the pulmonary edema and heart weakness. The temperature drops, and the mucous membranes become cyanotic.

The so-called diamond-skin disease (Fig. 5–6), characterized by regular rhomboidal lesions, sometimes appears in acute cases. In such an event, the affected swine die within 3 days after the onset of the disease. Such lesions on the skin are often associated, however, with a less severe type of swine erysipelas in which the symptoms are milder and rapidly subside after the appearance of the characteristic skin eruption. Unless complications set in, hogs affected with the mild type of erysipelas usually recover within 2 weeks. Where the diamond-skin lesions extend over considerable areas, however, there

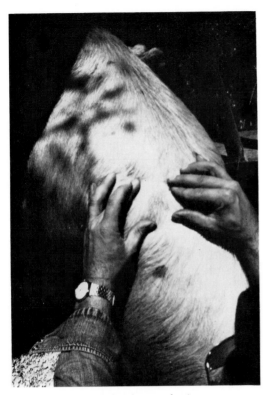

Fig. 5–6. Diamond-skin disease of swine.

may be a dry, gangrenous sloughing of large portions of skin. The ears and tail are often lost in this way. Loss of the tail, which is the more frequent occurrence, may be the only apparent evidence of past or present infection. Skin lesions are difficult to see except on light-colored breeds of hogs or on the light parts of dark breeds.

The swine that do not die of the disease are often left in a condition unprofitable to the owner. Many have swollen joints, and these animals are discounted by packer-buyers. Hogs that do not develop enlarged joints may become dehydrated and gaunt. These animals are often called race-horse pigs by owners because they eat a great deal but do not fatten as profitably as normal hogs. (Swollen joints may appear as an independent manifestation of the disease. All joints may be enlarged, but those of the knee, hock, and toes are most frequently affected.)

At times, the only indication of infection is a dry, scaly dermatitis, which is nonparasitic in character and fails to clear up in response to changes of feed or the application of parasiticides. As a rule, such lesions disappear upon the administration of specific antiserum, alone or in combination with living culture, or with antibiotic treatment.

Mortality is generally highest in the 1- to 3-month-old age group; but, again, all ages are susceptible. In the peracute cases, death may occur without noticeable signs. Most often, death occurs 3 to 7 days following the first signs of sickness. If the animal lives beyond that period, it either recovers or becomes a chronically infected carrier. Mortality is low among chronic carriers except in those affected with valvular endocarditis.

Subacute Erysipelas

This condition is less severe than the acute form. The swine do not appear ill; temperatures may not be as high or as long; appetite may be unaffected; skin lesions may appear but are less evident and easily missed; and, if visibly sick, the pigs do not remain so for the same length of time as do the acutely affected.

Chronic Erysipelas

This condition follows acute infection and is characterized by necrotic changes involving loss of portions of the skin, ears, tail, and feet. Valvular changes in the heart occur and, most importantly, arthritis is present.

The areas of necrotic skin are dark, dry, and firm; they eventually become separated from the healing underlying tissue and fall off, leaving an ugly scar. Secondary infection usually occurs and slows the healing process, which extends over many weeks.

Localization of the infection on the heart valves can cause cardiac insufficiency, which is most noticeable following exertion.

Chronic arthritis results in joints with various degrees of stiffness and enlargement. Interference with locomotion ranges from slight to complete, depending on extent of damage and number of joints involved. Apparently healthy pigs in affected herds may develop arthritis, in spite of treatment, at a later date. All chronic instances of swine erysipelas are the result of some degree of acute infection.

Acute nonsuppurative arthritis in lambs and calves is manifested by painful, slightly swollen hock, stifle, elbow, knee, and hoof joints. Although most animals recover in a few weeks, growth rate in young animals is adversely affected by their unwillingness to move about and graze. In a few lambs, the infection persists and causes permanent enlargement of the joints. Such animals are usually unthrifty and many are condemned when sent to slaughter.

Most outbreaks follow such traumatic events as castration, dehorning, and shearing. The erysipelas microorganism enters through skin wounds and localizes in the joints. The incubation period is constant, and lameness is noted 9 to 10 days following exposure.

Postdipping lameness is prevalent in older sheep and is an extension of infection that gains entry into the body through small cuts or abrasions on the feet and legs. These small wounds result from grass and wire cuts or from contact with the rough surface of the dipping vats. The erysipelas microorganism is a common contaminant and reproduces in most dipping solutions unless adequate amounts of copper sulfate are added. Once the bacteria gain entrance, the resulting infection spreads to the laminae of the hoof, causing acute pain and lameness.

Erysipeloid is a wound infection in human beings caused by E. rhusiopathiae. The incubation period is 2 to 5 days and is usually evidenced by a localized, swollen, hot, and painful lesion. In some animals the infection may extend to nearby joints, but in most occurrences there is no suppuration and inflammation subsides in a few days. In rare instances there may be a generalized septicemia accompanied by skin eruptions.

Postmortem Signs

In most instances, the microorganism causing swine erysipelas enters the body by way of the digestive tract. However, in a significant number of cases, the bacteria gain entry through the skin. Regardless of route of entry, the microorganisms multiply rapidly, and bacteremia results in less than 24 hours. The severity of the infection is determined by the degree of virulence of the bacteria and the resistance or susceptibility of the host.

Few pathologic lesions distinguish acute swine erysipelas from other septicemias, with the exception of individual skin lesions. Lymph nodes may be enlarged, the liver and spleen may be congested, and the mucosa of the stomach and small intestine may be slightly inflamed. If the joints are involved, the amount of fluid is increased and the tissue within the joint capsule may appear inflamed.

Swine afflicted with the chronic type of erysipelas have enlargement of one or more joints, with an increase in synovial fluid and thickening of the joint tissues. In severe cases, the joints may be calcified and ankylosed. A gangrenous process may involve the skin, the ears, the tail, and the feet. Many internal organs show evidence of chronic inflammation, and there are often vegetations on the heart valves; the localization of the microorganisms and the irritation they cause produce granulation tissue and fibrin, which adhere to the valves. Such vegetations often interfere with normal heart function and lead to the death of the host.

In instances of nonsuppurative polyarthritis in lambs and calves, postdipping lameness in sheep, and erysipeloid in man, the causative agent enters the body via a skin wound, rapidly multiplies, and causes a generalized bacteremia. As with swine, the severity of infection varies with the virulence of the bacteria and the resistance of the host; however, in most instances, there is extension of the infection with localization in the joints. The pathologic appearance of the affected joints is similar to that seen in swine.

Diagnosis

Diagnosis in the field is usually based on a history of sudden illness and other signs, prevalence of the disease in the area or on the farm, and postmortem findings.

The diagnosis of swine erysipelas presents difficulties, but in areas where it has become prevalent, veterinarians have been able to recognize it with a fair degree of accuracy through clinical observations supported by laboratory findings. At times, the disease is confusing, however, because it may appear in many ways.

Diagnostic signs are sudden onset, typical skin discoloration, dehydration, evidence of pain on moving, reluctance to move unless forcibly aroused, enlarged joints, eczema, sloughing of patches of skin, and high temperatures. The eyes may be clear and the squeal vigorous.

Specimens from suspected outbreaks of swine erysipelas may be forwarded to a diagnostic laboratory for bacteriologic examination. Generally, laboratory tests are considered to be more applicable to herd problems than to the diagnosis of the disease in individual animals. When erysipelas is suspected in a herd, a number of animals should be bled, and the diagnosis should be delayed until the representative serologic picture of the herd can be obtained. Remember that the chronic form of swine erysipelas may be present in a herd also affected with some other acute disease. A positive identification of the swine erysipelas bacterium does not rule out the possibility of another infection.

Control and Prevention

The biologic control of swine erysipelas may be attempted by several methods: (1) hyperimmune serum, (2) serum plus virulent culture of E. rhusiopathiae, or (3) avirulent or attenuated bacterins. The use of serum plus culture is not currently approved in all states; the serum-culture product is available only in states where swine erysipelas is common and disease-control authorities have authorized its use.

Hyperimmune serum may be used at any time in swine because there is no danger of spreading the disease by this means. Normal pigs injected with serum receive immediate passive immunity of about 2 weeks' duration.

Bacterins are safe because they do not infect other species of animals but do confer an immunity of relatively short duration. In most instances, this procedure is useful because the pigs are protected until they are marketed. When an outbreak occurs, doses of 10 to 30 ml of serum are used as early in the course of the disease as possible.

Live-culture strains of swine erysipelas bacteria of low virulence but high immunizing potential are currently used extensively in the United States in avirulent vaccines. An oral type of vaccine of low virulence is also available commercially. These vaccines usually provide immunity for as long as 1 year. Serum alone is effective only when given early in the acute stage of the disease; after the disease establishes itself and becomes chronic, the value of the serum is limited.

Swine erysipelas is difficult to eradicate because of the insidious and widespread distribution of the microorganism, its association with a wide variety of animals, and its ability to adapt to either a parasitic or saprophytic existence. The control of carrier animals is of utmost importance to the farmer, and no replacements should be brought onto a farm without a thorough knowledge of the herd of origin and without isolating the new animals for at least 30 days.

Animals should be maintained in uncontaminated areas under modern conditions of practical husbandry, where special attention is paid to housing, nutrition, sanitation, and immunization procedures. When an outbreak does occur, treatment should be initiated as quickly as possible, dead animals should be safely buried, exposed animals should be isolated, and the exposed area should be decontaminated before restocking with susceptible animals.

Treatment

Early treatment of acute swine erysipelas with immune serum and/or penicillin is effective. The response to treatment often occurs within 24 hours with complete elimination of clinical signs. The use of immune serum for reversal of signs is considered good evidence for diagnosis of the disease.

CHAPTER **6**
Diseases with Signs of Urinary and Genital System Changes

The urinary system consists of kidneys, ureters, bladder, and urethra. Alterations to these structures by obstruction (urolithiasis) or in the function by infection (leptospirosis) are accompanied by signs of pain and changes in the urine. The cause of each of these diseases, nutrition for water belly and infection for leptospirosis, is preventable. Vibriosis, brucellosis, and mastitis are infections of parts of the genitalia. Vibriosis, a venereal disease, and brucellosis, a systemic infection, affect reproduction. Mastitis, which is inflammation of the mammary gland, severely affects milk production and, potentially, the life of the animal.

RECOMMENDED READING

Amstutz, HE: Bovine Medicine and Surgery. 2nd Edition. Chaps. 4, 17, and 23. Santa Barbara, American Veterinary Publications, 1980.

Blood, NC, Henderson, JA, and Radostits, OM: Veterinary Medicine: A Textbook of the Diseases of Cattle, Sheep, Pigs and Horses. 5th Edition. Philadelphia, Lea & Febiger, 1979.

Hafez, ESE: Reproduction in Farm Animals. 4th Edition. Philadelphia, Lea & Febiger, 1980.

Philpot, WN: Mastitis Management. Oak Brook, IL, Babson Bros. Co., 1978.

Schalm, OW, Carroll, EJ, and Jain, NE: Bovine Mastitis. Philadelphia, Lea & Febiger, 1971.

Current Concepts of Bovine Mastitis. 2nd Edition. Washington, DC, National Mastitis Council Inc., 1978.

The Modern Way to Efficient Milking. Chicago, Milking Machine Manufacturers Council, 1979.

Water Belly

Water belly, or urolithiasis, is a noninfectious disease of cattle, sheep, and swine caused by the formation or lodging of concretions within the urinary tract. Urinary calculi are commonly found in feedlot cattle and sheep and are of greatest economic importance in feeder animals. In domestic animals, the condition may be found in either sex; the greatest clinical incidence is in steers and wethers, although bulls, rams, and females may also be affected.

Water belly is most frequently seen in feedlot cattle and sheep during the winter months, on full feed, in semiarid parts of the country where the mineral content of the water is high, and where animals are maintained on a heavily supplemented diet. In particular, feeds with high levels of calcium and phosphorus, such as legumes and cereal grains, and root fodders, such as beets, potatoes, and turnips, tend to lower the urine pH and induce the precipitation of ionic salts. Bacterial cells in the bladder, or desquamated epithelial or blood cells, may serve as nuclei for the deposition of dissolved salts when the urine pH changes. Excessive crystalline salt concentration occurs with inadequate water intake, high mineral intake, or associated urinary infections. Once deposition of salts around a nucleus has begun, the resulting calculus may serve as the framework for further deposition, and consequently, calculi may increase to a large size if undisturbed in the bladder. Most calculi, however, are small, varying in size from that of a grain of sand to that of a pea.

In females, the small gravel readily passes through the relatively large, short, unrestricted urethra and does not usually cause damage. Calculi remaining in the bladder, however, may increase in size appreciably and may eventually occlude the lumen of the urethra where it leaves the bladder.

In males, the calculi usually lodge at the sigmoid flexure of the penis, where further deposition, with inflammation and occlusion of the urethra, takes place. When males are castrated too early, the penis remains in an infantile condition and may not allow small gravel to pass with the normal urine. Estrogenic hormones in the feed of fattening steers may also predispose the animals to the retention of calculi in the urethra.

CAUSE

Water belly is caused by obstruction by concretions in the urinary tract, including the kidneys, ureters, bladder, and urethra. The contributing factors are complex but appear to be related to a deficiency of chloride and sulfate ions in the urine.

SIGNS

The signs of water belly, or urolithiasis, may vary in severity and appearance according to the location of occluding calculi. Animals suffering from advanced signs of this condition appear depressed and exhibit edema of the belly wall. If calculi form in the hilus of the kidney, there may be no signs of discomfort, especially if only one side is involved because the opposite kidney compensates for the loss of kidney function. If, however, a ureter becomes blocked, the animal exhibits intermittent pain. If the calculi lodge in the urethra, there is restlessness, reluctance to move, pain in the abdominal region, and depression. The temperature is elevated. The animal stamps its feet and strikes at the abdomen. Affected animals walk with a straddling gait, and stretch and attempt to urinate frequently with little or no success. An accumulation of fine gravel may be deposited on the preputial hairs, and the tail head is held high (Fig. 6-1). If the urethra is palpated over the ischiatic arch, it will be enlarged and pulsating, and if the bladder is palpated via the anus, it will be distended and tense.

With complete urethral obstruction, the animal cannot pass any urine; this leads to distension of the bladder and the abdomen. If not relieved, the bladder will rupture and the subcutaneous tissues of the lower abdomen will be infiltrated with urine, hence the name "water belly." Rupture of the bladder relieves the pain associated with this condition, but the distension of the abdomen with urine leads to uremia and eventually to death.

At autopsy, the principal findings are calculi occluding either the bladder outlet or the urethra, usually at the sigmoid flexure. The tissue around the site of the obstruction and extending back toward the bladder is inflamed, necrotic, and hemorrhagic. In the event of rupture, there is a noticeable rent in the bladder. The abdominal cavity contains considerable blood-tinged urine, and the lower abdominal wall is swollen and infiltrated with urine. After rupture of the bladder, the carcass cannot be used for human consumption because the meat emits a strong odor of urine when cooked.

PREVENTION

The only treatment for water belly is surgical removal of the offending occlusion before the bladder ruptures. After the signs appear, little can be done; therefore, prevention is the most economic course of

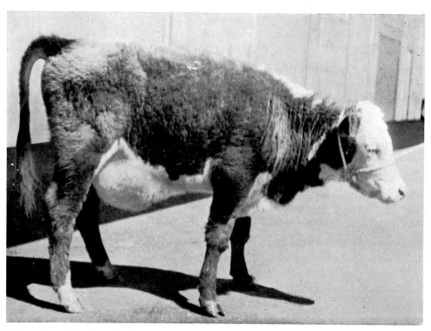

Fig. 6–1.   Distension of sheath and subcutaneous abdomen due to rupture of urethra. Note elevation of tail head. (From Gibbons, WJ: Clinical Diagnosis of Diseases of Large Animals. Philadelphia, Lea & Febiger, 1966.)

action. Some investigators have suggested that the disease may be prevented by adding salt in an amount up to 4% of the dry matter of the ration. The salt would cause the animal to drink considerable water, if available, and thus would tend to dilute the crystalline salts and wash them out with the urine. Others have recommended that the calcium and phosphorus ration be held to a 1:1 ratio and that adequate mineral-free water be available at all times. It is also suggested that castration be avoided until some genital development has taken place.

In consideration of preventive measures against urolithiasis, strict attention to diet must be emphasized. Rations high in sorghum grains, cottonseed hulls and meal, and molasses are conducive to the formation of calculi. In most semiarid areas where livestock are fattened in feedlots, the water usually is high in calcium and magnesium salts, which predispose to the formation of calculi. Under such circumstances, the use of ammonium chloride in the drinking water or in the diet protects cattle and sheep from urinary calculi. Ammonium chloride added to the diet at a rate of 1½ oz per steer, or ¼ oz for lambs, reduces the incidence of water belly to a low level. Calculi that form in lambs after treatment are small and usually pass easily in the urine. Calculi are seldom formed in steers after treatment.

Ammonium chloride is the best supplement found to date for lambs and cattle. Research will have to be conducted on other susceptible animals to determine whether this supplement will reduce the incidence of urinary calculi universally.

Leptospirosis

Leptospirosis is an infectious bacterial disease of cattle, swine, sheep, dogs, cats, rodents, wild animals, and man. The spirochetes causing the disease are enzootic in wild animals, which serve as natural reservoirs for the microorganisms. The disease may be transmitted from animal to animal and from animal to man, but progression usually stops with man.

Historically, the microorganisms causing leptospirosis were first seen in man in 1905, but the infective nature of the bacteria was not recognized until many years later. They were isolated from human beings who died following rat bites and were also found in the kidneys of rats. Leptospires were isolated from cattle in 1944 and from swine about 1950; however, the symptoms attributed to leptospires had been recognized for many years.

Geographically, the disease now known as leptospirosis has been diagnosed worldwide in domesticated livestock, in wild animals, and even in snakes. In the United States, leptospirosis is particularly widespread in cattle and swine.

CAUSE

Leptospirosis is caused by one or more serotypes of bacteria called Leptospira, the smallest of the spiral-shaped, slender rods called spirochetes. These cells are difficult to see and are visible only with the dark-field microscope or when special stains are used.

Serotype, rather than the usual "species" or "strains," is the term used to designate the subdivisions of the genus Leptospira. This variance from the usual classification is based on antigenic structure revealed by serologic investigations.

More than 120 serotypes have been found in the countries of the world. L. pomona, L. grippotyphosa, L. canicola, and L. icterohaemorrhagiae have been isolated from swine and cattle. In addition, L. hardjo and L. swajizak have been isolated from cattle. L. pomona and L. hardjo are common and are directly transmitted from animal to animal, whereas the others are less commonly transmitted from wildlife.

Leptospires are susceptible to drying, extremes of pH, and extremes of heat and cold; they do not withstand exposure to strong sunlight. They have low resistance to physical and chemical agents and are susceptible to iodine, calcium hypochlorite, and the cationic detergents.

TRANSMISSION

Carrier animals that have become urinary shedders after acute, mild, or, more often, inapparent infection serve as dangerous foci of infection. Direct infection results from contact with the urine of these shedders, whereas indirect transmission occurs when the bacteria are excreted into water or moist soil and susceptible animals subsequently come into contact with the contaminated environment.

Regardless of the serotype of Leptospira, or the species of animal involved, the signs produced are much the same except for variations due to individual resistance. The microorganisms gain entrance to the body through skin abrasions, through mucous membranes and conjunctiva via aerosols of infected urine splashed from hard surfaces or puddles, and through the intact skin.

Leptospirosis is spread to calves and piglets through the milk of infected dams. In adult animals, the microorganisms are primarily spread through contaminated feed and water. Animals are infected by drinking from ponds or sluggish, slow-moving streams contaminated by urine from barnyards or feedlots.

Arthropods have been incriminated as spreaders of leptospirosis, but they are not considered to be important vectors of the disease. The spirochetes are motile and may penetrate the unbroken skin of animals that have been exposed to contaminated water long enough for the skin to become softened.

Leptospires may survive for several weeks in the external environment with such optimal factors as mild weather, stagnant ponds and streams, and moist neutral soil of suitable chemical composition.

FACTORS INFLUENCING SUSCEPTIBILITY

In young animals, leptospirosis is often fulminating and fatal. In older animals, however, the disease is usually mild or inapparent. The disease occurs in all breeds and in both sexes. Age is the usual determinant of the severity of the signs. Young calves are usually infected by their dams. Piglets, on the other hand, are infected by rooting in heavily infected soil in barnyards or feedlots. Adult cattle are often infected by contact with the urine of swine on the same property. Lambs are commonly infected when they first begin to graze on contaminated pastures where either cattle or swine have been kept.

The disease may be spread from infected herd sires to susceptible females during the breeding season. A carrier animal provides a ready source of infection for young animals produced on the property and for suceptible replacements. Swine carriers may continue to shed viable leptospires in the urine for 6 months or more, whereas cattle may shed the bacteria for up to 3 months.

The season of the year, the climate, and the weather are not important as far as susceptibility is concerned. However, crowding animals into small areas and mixing animals of different ages do influence the spread of the disease.

CLINICAL SIGNS

The clinical signs and symptoms of leptospirosis vary considerably among species as well as among individuals within a species.

Leptospirosis in cattle is characterized by fever, prostration, jaundice, blood in the urine, abnormal milk, lowered milk production, and lack of appetite.

In swine, the signs of leptospirosis are mild and often inapparent. Abortions and the birth of weak pigs are the most obvious and often the only evidence of the disease.

Leptospirosis is usually divided into three forms—acute, mild, and chronic—depending on the severity and duration of the clinical signs.

The incubation period is relatively short, from 7 to 9 days. The acute form of the disease usually is seen in calves, is sudden in onset, and is fatal in 2 to 10 days; animals surviving this period usually recover, but their growth rate is retarded and they are slow to gain weight. The temperature rises to 105 to 107°F and persists for up to 56 hours. There is jaundice on the second or third day, and blood in the urine is followed by anemia. Because of the fever, there is lack of appetite and rapid loss of weight. Increased respiratory rate and difficult breathing are common signs.

The acute form is usually not as severe in adult cattle as in calves, although most of the clinical signs appear. In addition, however, lactating cows may develop bloody milk, with a dramatic drop in production, although the udder remains soft and pliable. Pregnant animals may abort at any stage of pregnancy, but most commonly during the last 3 months of gestation. Infected cows that recover usually produce dead or weak calves at term. Because the disease in older cattle is mild, the first suspicion of the disease may be associated with abortions in the herd or flock.

The mild form of leptospirosis, usually seen in older cattle, has similar but less severe signs. The temperature is not as high, and the observable signs may persist for only a few days. The only observable signs may be a slight drop in milk production and transitory blood in the urine.

In the chronic form of the disease, microscopic changes occur in the kidneys. Although abortion may occur during the last month of pregnancy, the usual sign is a mummified fetus or a weak calf at term. Retention of the fetal membranes following abortion is a common observance. Chronic loss of weight and persistent anemia are sequelae of this form.

The acute form of leptospirosis in swine is characterized by the small number of animals developing any clinical signs of disease. The infection spreads through a herd, as evidenced by serologic examination, but only a few animals are acutely ill at any one time. These animals demonstrate various levels of lack of appetite, fever, and diarrhea for a period of a few days.

In the chronic form in swine, the principal signs are abortion during the latter stages of gestation and birth of weak pigs at term. Metritis and lowered fertility have been associated with the disease, as have jaundice, anemia, hyperirritability, and transitory incoordination. Pigs farrowed at term but so devitalized that they die within a few hours are characteristic of this form of leptospirosis.

PATHOGENESIS AND POSTMORTEM SIGNS

Leptospires that enter the animal's body invade the circulatory system and rapidly multiply. Within 2 to 5 days, the microorganisms may be found in all organs and in the blood and urine.

Within 7 to 10 days, bacteria may be demonstrated with difficulty in the peripheral blood, but antibodies may be detected in the serum. After the appearance of antibodies, the spirochetes localize in the kidney tubules and continue to multiply; they are shed from the body in urine. During the time when the bacteria are rapidly multiplying in the blood, destruction of red blood cells causes hemoglobinuria, or red urine. At necropsy, there is generalized jaundice, anemia, and mottling of the liver. The kidneys appear swollen and congested, with small pinpoint hemor-

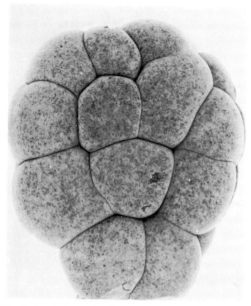

Fig. 6–2. Kidney of heifer affected with acute leptospirosis. (From Jensen, R, and Mackey, DR: Diseases of Feedlot Cattle. 2nd Edition. Philadelphia, Lea & Febiger, 1971.)

rhages covering their surface (Fig. 6-2). The bladder often contains dark-brown urine.

DIAGNOSIS

Diagnosis is usually based on clinical signs and herd history, but because of the similarity of other serious diseases, a differential diagnosis may be desirable. The most rapid method of diagnosis is an agglutination test using serum from an animal and prepared diagnostic antigens. Demonstrable antibodies first appear in the serum on about the sixth day of infection, and titers continue to increase during the active phase of the infection. As soon as the microorganisms are no longer shed via the urine, the serum antibody level declines to a more or less stable level and may persist for a year or more. Because bacterins and live attenuated cultures also result in persistent titers in the serum, a single positive serologic titer indicates only an exposure to the organisms or to the antibodies in colostrum or bacterins; it should therefore not be considered of di-

agnostic significance. Laboratory confirmation requires isolation of the organism from urine or infected or aborted fetuses.

CONTROL

Calves nursing cows that either have recovered from the clinical stages of this disease or have been vaccinated with a bacterin receive a degree of passive immunity lasting up to 2 months. The leptospiral antibodies are concentrated in the colostrum, and the calves usually demonstrate a higher antibody titer than do their dams.

Leptospirosis may be prevented, or at least controlled, by the judicious use of bacterins which, under favorable conditions, provide immunity for 6 months or more. Some animals, however, are afforded only partial immunity and become occult carriers of the disease unless they receive a second booster injection after an interval of 1 to 2 weeks. It is good policy to vaccinate all replacement animals added to a herd or flock and to vaccinate routinely all animals on a yearly basis.

Due to the peculiarity of the development of the disease in swine, sows should be vaccinated during the breeding season or after farrowing, but not during gestation; they should be revaccinated at each breeding season.

PREVENTION

Prevention of leptospirosis is based on breaking the cycle of transmission of bacteria and eliminating reservoirs of infection. The first step is to prevent contact of susceptible animals with infected urine. This may be achieved by sanitation, drainage of low swampy areas, and fencing of stagnant ponds and sluggish streams. Other husbandry methods include segregation of livestock by species and age groups, isolation of sick or aborting animals, and disinfection of all buildings or pens where sick or aborting animals have been housed.

All animals should be fed and watered under sanitary conditions to prevent contamination of racks, waterers, feed containers, feed, and water with urine from carriers. Most importantly, avoid feeding livestock on the ground.

All replacement or new animals must be isolated until they have passed 2 successive negative blood tests at least 30 days apart.

Some animals that have recovered from leptospirosis may be inapparent shedders of bacteria for varying periods of time.

Thus, all recovered animals should be isolated from healthy animals until laboratory tests reveal that they are no longer carriers of infection.

The most effective antibiotic seems to be dihydrostreptomycin, which at the level of 25 mg per kg of body weight helps to clear the infection. Because this antibiotic requires a long withdrawal period, its use in dairy herds is usually limited to those animals with clinical signs of the disease.

Vibriosis

The name of the organism causing vibriosis has been renamed Campylobacter fetus. The disease is still commonly referred to by its original name, which was derived from the former name of the organism, *Vibrio fetus*.

Vibriosis is an infectious disease of the genital tract caused by Campylobacter fetus var. venerealis and is characterized by infertility and occasional abortion. It is spread by breeding and is considered an important cause of infertility in cattle.

C. fetus var. venerealis is worldwide in distribution and was first described in this country in 1918. Because of the overshadowing importance of brucellosis at that time and the difficulty in culturing the organism, research progressed slowly. In 1940, however, infection was established as a cause of abortion and impaired breeding efficiency in affected herds. A few years later, scientists proved that venereal transmission resulted in delayed conception and irregular estrual cycles.

CAUSE

The disease is caused by the bacterium C. fetus var. venerealis. Isolated cultures have a short, comma shape but change to long, spiral-shaped filaments when cultivated artificially. Heat, light, and drying destroy the organism, but the sheep strain

can survive in soil, hay, and manure for several days.

C. fetus var. intestinalis does not affect cattle, but causes abortion in sheep and goats.

TRANSMISSION

Bovine campylobacter infection is usually transmitted through breeding, although it may be spread by artificial insemination with infected semen and by using contaminated instruments for examination. When naturally spread, the infection is evidenced primarily as temporary infertility with conception delayed 2 to 8 months. Some females have been known to carry the infection for at least 20 months. A few bulls become permanently infected, but all bulls may mechanically carry and spread infection.

Cattle of all ages seem to be susceptible, and spread is rapid in recently infected herds. Older animals usually throw off the infection eventually. Virgin heifers become infected upon exposure and maintain herd infection. Thus, the disease may remain a herd problem for years, with replacement animals, bulls, or carrier cows acting as reservoirs of infection. The infection rate in susceptible cows may approach 100%. In areas where cattle commonly mix on summer ranges or where infected cows or bulls have access to clean herds during the breeding season, the spread of disease is inevitable; clean bulls and virgin heifers are infected by carriers.

CLINICAL SIGNS

The usual effect of the disease is temporary infertility. At times, 16 services (with an average of 5) have been necessary to obtain a detectable pregnancy. In a field outbreak, few cows conceived on the first service from an infected bull. A low spring calving rate may be the first real evidence of the disease, and the calving period may be extended over the entire year.

The other prominent sign is the irregularity of the estrual cycle, which may range from 10 to 60 days. The long cycles occur as infection interrupts conception. The fetus is aborted or resorbed and a new cycle begins. If the fetus is expelled, it is often so small that it is overlooked, and the abortion is undetected. Any endometritis, vaginitis, and cervicitis sometimes produced may also be overlooked. Abortion rates of 4 to 29% have been reported. The abortions may occur at any stage of the gestation period but most happen in the fifth and sixth months.

The disease has no direct disabling effect on bulls; however, in infected herds with recurring estrus, bulls may become thin and emaciated through excessive breeding.

C. fetus causes a venereal disease that is transmitted by infected bulls to noninfected cows. The bacteria are deposited with the semen in the genital tract of the susceptible female. The organisms multiply and cause the death of the embryo in the first few weeks after fertilization. This occurrence is not followed by any signs of disease except the heifer's return to estrus. The infertility caused is temporary, and eventually, all animals recover. Some conceive as early as 2 months after exposure, but some remain infected for as long as 9 months. Six months after initial exposure, about 75% become pregnant if the bulls are

left with the cows. After recovery from the infection, cows have a measure of convalescent immunity to reinfection.

Most bulls are infected transiently, but are capable of spreading the infection for weeks after breeding an infected animal. Some bulls are permanently infected and carry the disease for years. Apparently, however, the cows that carry the infection are as important as the bulls in maintaining the disease from year to year in the herd. Carrier cows may give birth to normal calves in spite of infection.

DIAGNOSIS

The presence of Campylobacter infection may be suspected from the reproductive history and signs within the herd, but laboratory confirmation is desirable. The history may include introduction of animals from herds in which the disease or infertility is known to exist. Clinical tests to confirm a positive diagnosis include:

1. **Vaginal mucus agglutination test.** Vaginal mucus is absorbed on a sterile tampon. Then, in the laboratory, the mucus is extracted in saline and the agglutination test is performed.

2. **Isolation of C. fetus var. venerealis organisms from the bull.** This test is difficult because the organisms in semen or preputial washings are usually overgrown with contaminants. On the average, only one sample in five from known infected bulls is positive. In some instances, 15 consecutive samples have been required to find the organism.

3. **Isolation of C. fetus var. venerealis from the female genital tract.** Vaginal or cervical mucus is removed with a sterile pipette, and the organism is isolated by bacteriologic methods. This procedure is the most reliable. (The organism can also be isolated from the stomach of an aborted fetus.)

4. **Transmission test.** Suspect bulls are bred to virgin heifers. Then, the heifers are subjected to culturing techniques to recover and identify the organism.

CONTROL

Control measures may be instituted in noninfected herds by restricting replacements to virgin animals from known free herds. In infected herds, control may be accomplished by breeding a second herd of virgin animals to eventually replace the infected herd. (The replacement of infected cows in a year-round breeding program is inadvisable because it is expensive and impractical.)

Another method of control in infected herds is artificial insemination; this does not eliminate the disease, but does control further spread.

Usually the most practical and economical method of prevention and control is herd immunization with bacterin. A commercially produced adjuvant bacterin is so effective that pregnancy rates of 90% or higher have resulted in almost all infected herds treated with the bacterin.

Properly, the bacterin is used 30 to 120 days before breeding and possible exposure. Experiments have shown that active immunity is similar to convalescent immunity, and that both decrease with time. Revaccinating annually to maintain a level of immunity is economically sound. Of cows vaccinated 12 months prior to heavy exposure, only 56% were pregnant, whereas those bred to infected bulls following vaccination had a 70% pregnancy rate when rebred to infected bulls the second year. Infection and bacterin immunity complement each other, but infection cannot be depended on because most bulls lose the infection between breeding seasons. The vaccination of bulls is neither necessary nor desirable, for vaccinated bulls can continue to spread the disease mechanically. Pregnant animals can be vaccinated. Revaccination may be done at the usual weaning time, when the cows are being handled, without loss of efficiency.

An important cause of infertility in cattle can thus be controlled effectively by vaccination. The cost is low enough that many ranchers with clean herds are using vaccination to protect their herds from accidental infection from infected herds in the vicinity.

TREATMENT

The disease can be successfully treated with streptomycin. Although treating and clearing infected bulls for use on potentially infected cows is impractical, there are occasions when treating and clearing of infection from bulls to use on clean virgin heifers is feasible.

The disease in sheep and goats has been controlled and treated with some success by using a combination of feeding antibiotics and vaccination.

Brucellosis

Brucellosis is a contagious bacterial disease of cattle, swine, goats, sheep, man, and secondarily, of other animals. It is characterized by abortion, genital infection and the formation of localized lesions in various body tissues. Brucellosis is of public-health importance because of the debilitating disease (undulant fever) in man. All breeds of cattle are susceptible to the disease. The frequent occurrence of brucellosis in dairy cattle is associated with close housing and intensive management methods rather than with susceptibility factors. Likewise, the frequency in swine is due to foraging and eating habits rather than to particular susceptibility.

Brucellosis in goats is not a significant problem in this country. Sheep brucellosis has not been a problem in the United States, although it is a problem in some places in Europe.

Historically, brucellosis was recognized

as a contagious disease for many years before the causative bacteria were isolated. The Brucella microorganisms were first isolated in 1887 from human beings in the Mediterranean area, who were suffering from a malady known as Malta fever. Later, in 1905, the organisms were isolated from goat's milk and cheese in Malta, and were named Brucella melitensis. In 1897, B. abortus was isolated from aborted fetal membranes and fetal stomach contents in Denmark. Brucellosis of swine, formerly called contagious abortion of swine, was recognized as a specific disease when B. suis was isolated in 1914 in the United States. In 1930, a strain of B. abortus of low virulence but good immunizing properties was isolated and ultimately used to make Strain 19 bacterin, which is used to immunize young calves against the disease.

Geographically, brucellosis occurs in most swine-raising areas of the United States and in most countries of the world where swine exist in the domesticated or wild state. The disease is encountered in cattle throughout the world and is of major economic importance to cattle producers.

CAUSE

Although each class of livestock is primarily infected with a particular species of Brucella, each of the three Brucella species is capable of infecting human beings and any class of livestock. Thus, brucellosis must be considered as one disease-control problem for all livestock, not as three different control problems. All three species are related serologically, morphologically, and culturally.

B. suis is the primary cause of brucellosis in swine and is the species most often isolated from infected herds. However, B. melitensis and B. abortus are capable of causing infection in swine under natural conditions of exposure.

B. abortus is the principal cause of brucellosis in cattle, although the other species have been isolated on numerous occasions.

All species of Brucella that affect livestock are coccoid in shape, gram-negative, and have characteristic growth requirements. B. abortus requires increased carbon dioxide tension for isolation, whereas the others grow well under ordinary laboratory conditions. Although all species are similar, they exhibit individual differences to certain dyes.

All species are susceptible to pasteurization temperatures and quickly die when exposed to drying and direct sunlight. However, the bacteria are resistant outside the animal body when maintained in cool, moist surroundings. They have been found to remain viable in aborted fetuses at freezing or near-freezing temperatures for up to 824 days, although such conditions are seldom present under normal circumstances. The microorganisms are also susceptible to most common disinfectants if properly used.

TRANSMISSION

The bacteria causing brucellosis are shed in the milk, especially the colostrum, and in uterine discharges several days before abortion and up to several months following parturition. Some adult females may spread bacteria during the entire gestation period without exhibiting any other sign of the disease.

Brucellosis in cattle is commonly transmitted by close association with contaminated animals and environment. Fetuses and placental material resulting from abortion caused by brucellosis are heavily infected with the disease-causing bacteria and are readily available to any other susceptible animal. The contaminated material may remain infective for a long time, thus increasing chances of spread. Because Brucella commonly enters the body through the alimentary canal, the disease may be spread by animals licking the genital organs or the placenta or vaginal discharge of an infected animal. The conjunctiva and mucous membranes of the nose, as well as the vagina, provide for convenient entry. Infection may also result from the ingestion of contaminated grass, water, and dry roughage.

Transmission from bull to cow during natural service has been demonstrated; however, this route of infection is rare unless the bull is shedding viable bacteria in the semen. Semen from a contaminated bull used for intrauterine artificial insemination is a common source of infection.

Swine brucellosis is transmitted chiefly by direct contact. Therefore, an infected animal from a new herd can spread the disease into the herd to which it is introduced. An animal may become a carrier if it comes in contact with carriers at a show or fair.

The disease is transmitted from boar to female during natural service. Ingestion of the products of abortion, food and water contaminated with vaginal exudates of infected and aborting females, milk from infected sows or gilts, or other infected material is an easy means of entry into the alimentary canal.

Young animals born to dams that are carriers are covered with viable bacteria and may spread the disease through a crowded barnyard. Calves and piglets nursing from infected dams may spread the bacteria throughout an area with their feces, particularly if unconfined.

It is often difficult to discover how brucellosis has gained entry into a herd. However, the infected female, usually a healthy carrier, is the most common vector for spread, both within the herd and from herd to herd. Precautions must be exercised to insure that new animals introduced into a herd are free of brucellosis. New animals should be quarantined and tested to be sure that they were not incubating the disease at the time of purchase.

Dogs, birds, and feral animals may occasionally be incriminated as spreaders of brucellosis by dragging infected, aborted fetuses from one property to another. Improperly cleaned vehicles used to transport animals may be sources of infection for susceptible animals, as may unsanitary sales barns, show rings, and holding yards.

FACTORS INFLUENCING SUSCEPTIBILITY

Season of the year, climate, and weather apparently are of little significance as factors of suceptibility to brucellosis. Age and sex, however, are important. Although all males are susceptible to infection, bulls appear to be quite resistant, whereas boars are very susceptible to brucellosis. Females are much more susceptible than males, but all females are not equally susceptible. Some are naturally immune and resist infection even if exposed to a massive dose of bacteria. Some have moderate immunity, and others have none.

Young calves and piglets appear to have a natural resistance to brucellosis and seldom become infected, although they may harbor the bacteria temporarily and spread viable microorganisms in their feces until weaned. In some instances, young animals have been infected at birth and have carried the microorganisms until maturity, at which time the usual signs appeared. In most instances, the fetus infected in utero, however, loses the infection before reaching 6 months of age. Brucellosis may, therefore, be considered a disease of mature animals.

The progress of the disease depends on the individual. Most animals are readily able to resist the disease before reaching sexual maturity, but as they approach maturity, their susceptibility increases. Sexually mature bulls seem more resistant than sexually mature heifers or cows. Pregnant cattle are more apt to get the disease than are nonpregnant cattle, and their disease is more severe.

CLINICAL SIGNS

Of the primary signs of brucellosis in cows, the act of abortion is the most characteristic, although all infected pregnant animals do not necessarily abort. In addition to abortion, the birth of weak calves, retained placenta, and vaginal discharge are prevalent signs. Any of these may be followed by temporary infertility. In animals infected while open, signs are generally absent. The prominent signs in infected bulls generally are enlargement of one or both testicles, loss of sexual desire, and infertility (Fig. 6-3). These signs are usually accompanied by infection of one or more of the accessory sex organs, which can be determined only by rectal examination.

If an animal has some resistance, or if the infection is of low virulence, the disease has a tendency to localize, without clinical signs, in the udder or its lymph glands; in these instances, the bacteria may persist for life, reappearing in the uterus during pregnancies.

Usually, the first suspicion of brucellosis in a herd is unexplained abortion or return to service by a previously bred female. The disease is insidious in its manifestations, and the signs of impending abortion are no different from those of normal parturition, except that they may occur at any time during the gestation period, depending on the time of infection. Some females may abort early without any warning signs, although usually the abortion occurs during the latter stages of pregnancy.

The incubation period is variable and depends on the age of the female and the stage of pregnancy at which infection occurred. The younger the fetus at the time

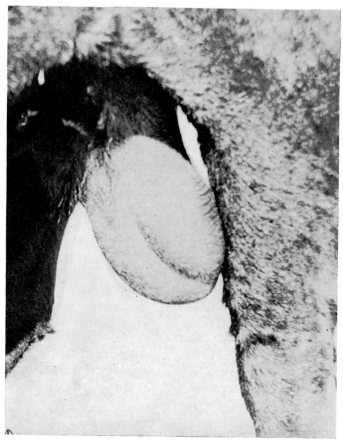

Fig. 6–3. Orchitis in bull due to brucellosis. (From Gibbons, WJ: Clinical Diagnosis of Diseases of Large Animals. Philadelphia, Lea & Febiger, 1966.)

of infection, the longer the incubation period. During experiments, when the exact time of infection was known, abortions occurred at varying lengths of time after 2 weeks of incubation.

The establishment of a carrier state in cows may be associated with a reduction in milk production, dead calves at term, retained placenta, and metritis. Also, in this chronic stage of the disease, there may be lameness due to accumulations of bacteria in joint capsules, causing swelling and pain. In the male, there may be enlargement, hardening, and even abscess formation in the testes, with resultant pain and lowered sexual drive.

The classic clinical manifestations of B. suis infection are abortion, birth of stillborn or weak pigs, infertility, unilateral or bilateral orchitis, posterior paralysis, and lameness. Decreased sexual drive is occasionally observed in affected boars.

Abortions have been observed as early as 22 days following natural service to boars disseminating B. suis in the semen. Early abortions are usually overlooked under field conditions, and the first indication of infection is a large percentage of sows or gilts showing signs of estrus 30 to 45 days after service terminating in conception. Little or no vaginal discharge is observed with early abortions. Abortions during the middle or late stages of gestation usually occur in females that acquire infection after pregnancy has advanced past 35 or 40 days. The persistence of genital infection in females varies considerably. B. suis usually persists for a minimum of 1 month in the nongravid uterus. In a group of sows bred to boars disseminating B. suis in the semen, several shed the microorganism in vaginal discharge for at least 30 months. An apparently abnormal vaginal discharge is seldom observed in sows with uterine infection. The percentage of females eventually recovering from genital infection is relatively high.

Infection of cattle with B. suis is rare; it is usually localized in the udder or nearby lymph nodes with no clinical signs. There is little information on B. melitensis in cattle, but limited studies show that it causes udder and uterine infection with occasional abortion.

PATHOGENESIS

After they invade the body, the microorganisms enter the blood and are carried to various organs and tissues where they multiply freely. The udder, uterus, testicles, seminal vesicles, lymph glands, and spleen are most often affected. Abscess formation is common in affected organs and tissues.

During pregnancy, the microorganisms localize in the superficial inguinal lymph nodes and udder and then infect the placenta and fetal fluids. They localize in the epithelial cells of the chorion, where they cause necrosis and eventual death of the fetus and subsequent abortion. The appearance of the placenta is leather-like, thickened, and brownish in color, with marked necrosis of the cotyledons. After or just prior to abortion, bacteria appear in the mammary glands and their lymph nodes.

In bulls and boars, bacteremia results from localized infection of the seminal vesicles, testes, and epididymis. In many males the infection becomes chronic, leading to permanent destructive changes in the testes and to infertility.

DIAGNOSIS

The diagnosis of brucellosis is based on isolation of infective bacteria from the vaginal exudates of aborting females, from the tissues of aborted fetuses, from semen of infected males, and from the milk of lactating females. The field diagnosis may be made by one or more diagnostic screening laboratory tests, followed by serologic examination for antibodies. A rising titer is significant in adult animals, but of little value in positive diagnosis in immature animals that may have received antibodies transferred from the dam in milk.

CONTROL

Viable bacterins have been shown to be of value in the control of brucellosis in cattle, but have been of little use in combating the disease in swine. When coupled with a program of test and slaughter, calfhood vaccination has been of value in eradication programs in this country.

In 1930, scientists in the U.S. Department of Agriculture isolated a strain of Brucella characterized by low virulence and high antigenic properties, called Strain 19, now used on a worldwide basis.

Calfhood vaccination with B. abortus Strain 19 vaccine (bacterin) is effective in increasing resistance to the disease. However, resistance is not complete in all instances (because of individual differences) and breaks to some extent in the presence of massive exposure. In most calves, the immunity does not decline with the passage of time. Caution must be exercised, however, in the use of the vaccine because some calves carry a persistent titer into adult life. This causes confusion because the difference between a vaccination titer and a frank infection titer is difficult to determine. Most young calves lose the vaccination titer by the time of sexual maturity although the immunity persists for life.

PREVENTION

Calfhood vaccination, intensive application of milk-ring and serologic tests in a manner prescribed by governmental regulatory agencies, are used to combat brucellosis on a nationwide basis. These procedures must be coupled with sanitary measures aimed at preventing contact of susceptible animals with infected animals and material.

A national cooperative swine brucellosis eradication program is based on a voluntary herd-validation program.

The state-federal cooperative plan for the eradication of brucellosis in cattle is one of the most important regulatory programs now in operation in this country. The dairy industry is responsible for persistent calfhood vaccination, annual testing of adult cattle, and accurate maintenance of records to sell milk on the open market and to obtain the coveted "Certified Brucellosis-Free" status.

There are several options by which "Certified Brucellosis-Free" status may be obtained, but to be retained, all herds must be tested according to USDA rules and regulations as set forth in *Recommended Uniform Methods and Rules—Brucellosis Eradication*. This publication may be obtained from state or federal veterinarians or from local accredited veterinarians.

Currently, 30 states are qualified as certified brucellosis-free areas. Herds in the other 20 states account for 97% of the newly infected herds in the United States during 1979. During the first two quarters of 1980, there was an alarming increase in the number of newly infected herds in both certified and noncertified states.

The *Uniform Methods and Rules for Brucellosis Eradication* have been strengthened to better control interstate movement of infected cattle. Effective January 1, 1982, there is further restriction of the movement of cattle within and between states. State classifications were changed to A, B, or C status. Class A states must have had no infected herds for 12 months. Cattle from Class A states may move out of state without a blood test. Class B states must have a herd infection rate of less than 1%. No county within a Class B state can have an annual herd infection rate of over 2%. In order to move cattle from a Class B state, a negative test must be obtained within 30 days before shipment and another negative test 45 to 120 days after movement. Both Class A and Class B states must have effective surveillance programs. Cattle in Class C states (over 1% annual herd infection rate) must obtain 2 negative tests at 60-day intervals prior to movement and another negative test 45 to 120 days after movement.

In addition to more stringent control of cattle movement, more stringent rules to provide identification of cattle and changes in vaccination dosage are being adopted. At the time of this writing, brucellosis eradication in the United States is not a reality. The infection of cattle in southeast and south central regions of the United States remains to be satisfactorily controlled.

Mastitis of Dairy Cows

It has been said that mastitis is a disease of man manifested in dairy cows. This is a tongue-in-cheek exaggeration, but its implication is not completely in error. It implies that man is responsible and can control the disease. When the economic importance of mastitis in beef cattle is compared with that in dairy cattle, it is obvious that the development of cows to lactate far in excess of normal needs has created problems. It is estimated that production lost to mastitis in dairy cows exceeds 1 billion dollars per year in the United States at current values. The beef industry does not consider losses to mastitis as significant. Man has tampered with nature and developed a highly productive but sensitive gland susceptible to infection. Additionally, man has established facilities and production units to remove milk from the gland in the most expedient, efficient, and profitable manner. So, man is in control, but complete control over all the factors causing mastitis is difficult.

The term "mastitis" means inflammation of the mammary gland. It comes from a Greek word *mastos* for breast and *itis* for inflammation. Injury to the tissue results in inflammation. The extent of damage to milk-producing tissue depends on the type and extent of injury. The process of healing may restore all the tissue to function, one part may be functional and one part may be destroyed, or all parts may be destroyed. If the injured tissue becomes infected, it may be cleared by natural defense mechanisms, a chronic status may develop, or it may extend to a systemic infection endangering the cow's life.

SIGNS

Subclinical Mastitis

The signs of mastitis as manifested in dairy cows range from mild to severe. Sometimes there are no visible signs of the infection that is present. This type of mastitis, which is called "subclinical," is detected only by changes in the milk constituents. The milk appears to be normal, and the udder is not swollen or changed in appearance. But the milk constituents are altered to have increased numbers of cells (leukocytes and tissue cells); less casein, lactose, and fat; and increased lipase, sodium, and chloride. These changes indicate mastitis and also reduce the value of milk. In addition to the changes in constituents, pathogenic bacteria are usually present. Streptococcus agalactiae and Staphylococcus aureus account for 90 to 95% of the causes of subclinical mastitis. This unseen type of change results in enormous loss of milk production and milk quality.

The presence of subclinical mastitis can be determined by testing the milk for the changes that have taken place. Many types of tests have been devised. Most are based on detecting the number of cells present in the milk. The number of cells present is directly proportional to the degree of inflammation and destruction of secretory tissue and lost milk production. Over 100,000 cells per milliliter is considered abnormal. Milk with more than 1.5 million cells per milliliter is considered unfit for human consumption and is not permitted for marketing. The number of cells can be estimated by such tests as the California mastitis test (CMT). This test consists of adding to milk a reagent that reacts with cells to cause a varying degree of gel. The thicker the gel formed, the more cells present. Cells can be accurately counted by the Direct Microscopic Somatic Cell Count (DMSCC) or by an electronic counter. Extensive worldwide studies show that lost milk production is 3% for cell counts of 150,000 to 225,000; 5% for 260,000 to 380,000; 8 to 12% for 420,000 to 1.2 million; and 16 to 26% for 1.28 to 2.28 million cells per milliliter. The cell counts of milk from most herds range from 420,000 to 790,000 cells per milliliter. This indicates approximately a 10% reduction in potential milk production caused by subclinical mastitis.

Clinical Mastitis

If the inflammatory reaction is severe enough, the changes can be seen. The milk may contain flakes or clots of debris resulting from tissue damage, or the milk may be thin and watery indicating that milk secretory cells have been damaged. Some reactions are severe enough to cause swelling of the affected quarter. In addition to the swelling, there is evidence that the quarter is painful and hot. A still more severe reaction produces signs that indicate that the disease has affected the cow as well as the mammary gland. In addition to the changes in the milk and the swelling of the gland, the cow stops eating and has a fever. In extreme instances, usually associated with a coliform infection, the cow is dull, weak, and shows signs of toxicity and dehydration. The gland may be so severely affected that it becomes cold and gangrenous. Death is not uncommon when the infection produces such a severe toxemia.

THE COW AND HER DEFENSES

The hazards imposed on the gland by man's system to harvest milk are many and varied. The type of cow that has been developed is not an agile, graceful creature, but is large bodied, awkward, and subject to the stresses of metabolism that convert high-energy rations to more than her body weight in milk production each month. The mammary gland converts blood to milk at a ratio of approximately 400 parts blood to 1 part milk. This gland, with its rich and extensive blood supply and delicate secretory tissue, is exposed to ground contamination and bruising each time the cow lies down. The act of a cow rising from recumbency is not a fluid graceful movement. Hopefully the cow can accomplish this act without tangling the udder with her own claws. The cow must endure the close proximity of other cows and hope to avoid being stepped on. She must travel the lanes or routes established to get from pasture or holding pen to feed bunk and milking parlor without injury. She must endure whatever climatic conditions prevail. She must withstand the process of being milked twice a day, which, if nothing else, involves a machine pulsating on each teat 500 times a day. And, she must endure the exposure to all the microorganisms that build up in the environment of a concentrated group of animals and their waste.

The cow and her mammary gland need protection to avoid mastitis. To protect her, the dairyman must understand and take advantage of her natural defense mechanisms and must understand and control the microorganisms that may cause mastitis. The size and shape (conformation) of the mammary gland are influenced by heredity. It is no accident that some glands are wide and held snugly against the abdomen whereas others are pendulous. Careful selection results in development of glands less vulnerable to injury. Teat placement, shape, and length are also heritable characteristics. Ideally placed and sized teats conform to the twice daily use of a milking machine without injury and also are least vulnerable to injury in the environment. Long, narrow teats are easily stepped on, pulled too far into the inflation during milking for adequate pulsation relief, and cause "squawking" from air entering the teat cup. Short, stubby teats require the teat cup to be pushed against the base causing constriction at the annular fold. Teats with everted or inverted ends are hard to clean. Large thin-walled teats have short, weak streak canals, thereby affording little protection to infection.

Although the skin covering the mammary gland, if unbroken, prevents the underlying tissue from becoming infected, the opening at the teat end is a potential point of entrance. The opening is designed to prevent infection. Milk from secreting cells moves through a system of branching ducts to collect in a cistern at the base of the teat and then to the teat cistern. Milk leaves the gland through a specialized canal leading to the opening. This is called the streak canal or teat canal. The canal is lined with stratified squamous epithelial cells that produce keratin. Keratin helps to seal the opening and is somewhat bactericidal. Surrounding the streak canal are muscle cells that help to close the opening. The canal dilates with let-down and the resulting internal pressure but requires several hours after milking to close tightly again. Some of the keratin lining is washed away during milking, but it rebuilds. If a cannula or teat infusion tube is threaded into the canal, most of the protective keratin is removed.

In addition to the mechanical protection at the teat opening, the reaction to an organism entering the mammary gland results in a mobilization of leukocytes (white blood cells) to engulf or destroy the organism. Leukocytes are always present in normal milk but increase rapidly when the mammary gland is inflamed or infected.

CAUSE

Anything that happens to the cow and her mammary gland to compromise the natural defense or protective mechanisms predisposes the animal to infection. Any situation that places a potential destructive organism (pathogen) in a position to enter the gland also predisposes the animal to infection.

There are many potential pathogens. The most common pathogens to cause mastitis are: Streptococcus agalactiae, Staphylococcus aureus, Streptococcus dysgalactiae, Streptococcus uberis, and a group called coliforms. If these organisms could be kept out of the mammary gland, mastitis losses would be minimal.

What is the nature of these organisms? Streptococcus agalactiae lives and multiplies in milk and mammary tissue. These organisms are shed in milk from infected cows and contaminate whatever they contact—milkers' hands, cloths, sponges, milking equipment, pipelines, bulk tanks, and the floor of the barn. Staphylococcus aureus lives and grows in the tissue of infected udders. It can also survive on the skin of milkers' hands and on utensils. Human strains of S. aureus can be transferred from the hands of milkers to cows and cause severe mastitis. Streptococcus dysgalactiae and S. uberis both live outside the cow and contaminate teats. Because these organisms do not require udder tissue or milk to survive, they are difficult to eradicate. Coliform organisms exist in manure and the environment contaminated with manure. Klebsiella, a coliform, lives on vegetation, tree bark, and wood and, therefore, is in wood shavings and sawdust.

PREVENTION

A complete list of all the possible predisposing causes and potential pathogens would probably discourage anyone from trying to prevent mastitis. However, there are some guidelines to consider:

1. Select replacement animals according to udder attachment and shape and teat size and placement.

2. Do not feed mastitic milk (Streptococcus agalactiae) to heifer calves, and do not let calves nurse each other.

3. Keep pastures free of wire, machin-

ery, junk, and any object that might injure a mammary gland.

4. Fence off ponds or swamp areas in pastures where cows might congregate or stand in hot weather.

5. Select well-drained pastures or control maternity stalls and lots for calving so cows are not contaminated by filth and manure.

6. Arrange traffic patterns so that cows do not cross ditches or climb rocks or slippery inclines to get to feeding or milking facilities.

7. Place feed bunks and water tanks on concrete or ground that does not become mush when it rains.

8. Arrange holding pens, free-stall alleys, and feeding platforms for manure removal by flushing or scraping.

9. Discourage cows from lying near the feed bunk by providing shelter sufficient to cover the feed but not to shade or protect the cows.

10. Maintain clean *dry* bedding in free stalls. If shavings or sawdust are used, it must be kept dry.

11. If a wash sprinkler system is used in the parlor holding pen, allow time for cows to drip dry before entering the milking parlor. When the underside of a cow remains dripping wet during preparation and milking, all the organisms on the outside of the cow drain down over the udder and toward the teats.

12. Prepare the udder for milking by using a fine, warm, water spray and dry thoroughly with *single-service paper towels*. Sponges, cloths, or rags carry live organisms from one cow to another even if soaked in disinfectant for several hours. S. agalactiae has been found in sponges as long as 7 days after the last use.

13. Strip several streams of milk (either into a strip cup or directly into a drain) from each quarter before applying the machine. This assures let-down, removes residual bacteria from the teat, and permits observation of the milk for clots or flakes or other changes.

14. Attach the claw without allowing it to snap on the teats and without allowing excess air to enter the teat cups. Air entering the claw can cause vacuum fluctuation in the system, thereby causing reverse jetting of milk droplets in claws attached to other cows.

15. Remove the machine when the udder is milked out by *first shutting off the vacuum*. Removal by allowing air into one teat cup causes reverse jetting; forcibly taking them off causes teat damage and sore teat ends. Do not machine strip except for individual slow milking quarters. Machine stripping is not harmful if done correctly, but it has been proved unnecessary and wastes time.

16. Dip teats with an effective germicidal teat dip immediately after removal of the milker. Most commercial teat dip solutions are effective (except those containing oils). Dip solutions containing some glycerin or lanolin are nonirritating and effective. Do not mistake sanitizing solutions for teat dips—one dipping with solutions designed to sanitize equipment can create sore teats and mastitis. The postmilking teat dip removes the last drop of milk and all the organisms from the skin of the teat that might migrate into the opening before it closes and seals. It also provides some protection against further contamination for the period between milkings.

17. Feed cows after milking. When cows are accustomed to going to the feed bunk after milking, they are not as likely to lie down during the hour or so required for the teat opening to close tightly.

18. Rinse the teat cups with sanitized solutions between cows. This can be done (with the vacuum shut off) by dipping two teat cups at a time in a bucket of disinfectant solution or by using the wash nozzle and spraying the disinfectant solution into the teat cups. Some systems have equipment designed to back-flush the claw and teat cups after each cow is milked. The objective of these procedures is to prevent the spread of infection from cow to cow.

19. Monitor the entire milking system by continuous maintenance and periodic inspections by qualified personnel to assure proper function, adjustment, and efficiency for both sanitizing and milking.

CONTROL

Achieving prevention is difficult and may be unrealistic, but if the goal is anything less, the end result will be unsatisfactory. Until the knowledge and means of eliminating all the causes are available, efforts to control and reduce losses are imperative. Intensive investigation of all facets of mastitis has been taking place for decades and is still occurring. Milking-equipment manufacturers are continuously improving systems and equipment as new knowledge surfaces. Microbiologists continue to search for a means of developing immunity to the common pathogens. Researchers continue to clarify the function of the mammary gland and its defense mechanisms. Trials are being conducted to develop ways to protect the teat from injury. Such organizations as the International Milk Federation and the National Mastitis Council sponsor programs and research to find better means of prevention and control. Milk marketing and manufacturing organizations are encouraging quality milk production by incentive bonuses to dairy farmers.

Several definite factors have emerged as essential for mastitis control.

1. Sanitation for the cows during and between milkings.

2. Drying the teats and udder before milking.

3. Dipping the teats with an effective germicidal solution after milking.

4. Correct installation, adjustment, and maintenance of equipment.

5. Proper milking technique.

6. Treatment of cows at drying-off with special-formula antibiotic infusions.

These factors, used in several large surveys involving herds in the United States, Great Britain, and Australia, proved to be effective in reducing mastitis levels and incidence by as much as 50% over a period of several years.

TREATMENT

Some mild infections of the mammary gland spontaneously disappear without treatment. Medicines are often given credit for what natural processes do. However, it is not safe to assume that a clinical case, without treatment or with minimal treatment, has been cured simply because the milk appears normal. Most clinical cases are flare-ups of a subclinical infection. It is estimated that there are 40 subclinical infected cows in a herd for every clinical case. The method of determining the effectiveness of treatment or whether an udder is free of infection is by having milk samples tested and cultured by a laboratory.

Treatment of a cow acutely sick from mastitis must be directed toward saving the cow's life. Antibiotics and detoxifying fluids and medications must be administered into the blood for rapid effect. Intramammary infusions of antibiotics following removal of all the debris and secretions may not be effective. The selection of the most likely effective antibiotic for treatment is essential. This treatment may require many days. A milk sample taken immediately and cultured and tested for sensitivity helps to determine the most effective antibiotic.

All clinical cases should be treated as they occur. The bacteria and cells in the milk from one infected cow can contaminate a tank of milk to an unacceptable level. Cows with milder clinical infections respond to intramammary infusion of antibiotics. Again, the antibiotic is selected according to the identity and sensitivity of the organism cultured from a milk sample. If samples are not collected before treatment is given, organisms will not grow on the laboratory media. Streptococcus infections, especially S. agalactiae, respond well to penicillin. Staphylococcus aureus infections do not respond well during lactation. Because Staphylococcus grows in the tissue, it may become walled off and form small abscesses that are difficult for medications to reach. Staphylococcus infections frequently become chronic, and the cows must be considered as dangerous carriers eligible for culling. Some may respond better to treatment during the dry period when the drug stays in contact longer and the gland is inactive.

There are two general precautions about treatment:

1. Home-made combinations of antibiotics should not be infused into udders. Contaminants in such concoctions have been responsible for more infections than the medicine was intended to cure.

2. Milk must be discarded from any cow under treatment, no matter how the drugs are given or which drugs are used. Antibiotics have different clearance times. All commercial infusion tubes are labeled as to how long to withhold milk. If strict adherence to withdrawal times for milk is not followed, a tank of milk may have to be discarded.

CHAPTER 7

Diseases with Signs of Changes on the Skin and the Mucous Membranes

This chapter discusses infectious, contagious diseases that cause noticeable lesions on the surface of the skin and mucous membranes. All these diseases are debilitating and cause losses in production. Control is difficult because of the ease of transmission.

RECOMMENDED READING

Amstutz, HE: Bovine Medicine and Surgery. 2nd Edition. Chaps. 12, 13, 21. Santa Barbara, CA, American Veterinary Publications, 1980.

Blood, DC, Henderson, JA, and Radostits, OM: Veterinary Medicine: A Textbook of the Diseases of Cattle, Sheep, Pigs, and Horses. 5th Edition. Philadelphia, Lea & Febiger, 1979.

Jensen, R: Diseases of Sheep. Chap. 6. Philadelphia, Lea & Febiger, 1974.

Infectious Papillomatosis (Warts)

Infectious papillomatosis, or common warts, is a disease occurring in cattle, goats, dogs, rabbits, and, sometimes, man in various parts of the world. The disease is characterized by the formation of warts, which are in effect benign tumors consisting of fibrous cores covered to a variable depth with stratified squamous epithelium, the outer layers of which become hyperkeratinized. The papillomas, or warts, occur as single, flower-like vegetations ranging in size from a pinhead to a large cauliflower 6 to 7 inches across. The vegetations may occur singly, in groups, or diffusely.

Historically, infectious papillomatosis has been known for centuries, but until the turn of this century research was not undertaken on this disease. Shortly thereafter, it was reported that warts from cattle could be transmitted to humans; this has not been substantiated, however. In 1929, it was discovered that papillomatosis could be transmitted from one animal to another, but only within the same species.

CAUSE

Infectious papillomatosis is believed to be caused by one or more viruses possessing a high degree of host specificity. However, interspecies transmission does not occur under usual conditions, although experimental transmission between species has been reported. The filterable viruses can be isolated from the vegetative growth on the skin of infected animals. The microorganisms can be cultivated on chick embryo tissue culture, and a vaccine has been made from agents grown by this method.

The exact mode of transmission of infectious papillomatosis is not known; however, it is thought to be transmitted by direct contact from an infected animal to a noninfected animal through small abrasions on the skin. There is further evidence that indirect transmission of the virus may occur through improperly cleaned bleeding needles and instruments used by careless herdsmen. It is believed that the virus gains entrance through small injuries in the skin and by direct contact of the injured areas with infected animals, and that it is transmitted indirectly from animal to animal by means of halters, nose leads, leashes, and other articles contaminated by contact with diseased animals. Indirect transmission may also result through contaminated hands of attendants and contaminated instruments of restraint. Biting insects may also play a role.

FACTORS INFLUENCING SUSCEPTIBILITY

Infectious papillomatosis is most often seen in calves and young cattle under 2 years of age, although adult bovine animals may become infected. In goats, the disease is most prevalent in animals over 1 year of age. The disease appears more frequently among stabled animals than among those allowed access to pasture or range. Because transmission is favored by direct contact, the condition is often seen in several animals in the same pen, whereas other animals of the same age in different pens nearby may not be affected. The incidence within a single pen, however, is variable; extensive numbers of warts are found on some animals and none on others. There is no relationship between the disease and sex, condition of the animal, or feeding practices.

CLINICAL SIGNS

Infectious papillomatosis may occur singly or in clusters. The lesions may be hard or soft elevated masses. Many warts are small and rounded, whereas others are broad, thin, long, or club shaped. Some warts become cauliflower-like growths, 6 to 7 inches across. These large growths are usually soft and give off a distinctive, offensive odor.

The warts are most frequently seen on the sides of the head, under the chin, and around the eyes, neck (Fig. 7-1), dewlap, and shoulder of young cattle, but seldom on the legs. When a calf is infected with a large number of warts, or when a few warts become excessively enlarged, the animal usually becomes unthrifty. Large warts are soft in nature and, thus, are easily injured. As most warts receive a plentiful blood supply from the skin, they bleed easily when injured, and the open wounds may become infested with parasites or contaminated by infective bacteria.

Warts may slough off spontaneously, and sometimes a new wart forms where an earlier wart had disappeared; however, most animals are resistant to further infection once an initial infection has regressed. If warts become too large, they may break off at the base and become necrotic. The necrosis serves as an irritant that aids in the sloughing-off process.

POSTMORTEM SIGNS

Infectious papillomas are benign tumors consisting of a fibrous core covered with stratified squamous epithelium. Upon postmortem examination, animals affected with an extensive infestation of warts show whitish cauliflower-like masses on the skin. In some adult dairy cattle, warts may be found in the teat canal, and in bulls, the disease may produce a fibrous papilloma on the penis or prepuce. Growths are often seen on the vulva and in the vagina of heifers, but whether this particular condition is related to infectious papillomatosis is doubtful. Warts are occasionally seen on the teats of cattle and are relatively distinct, invariably hard and cornified, and grayish or black in color. Warts may be sufficiently numerous on the udder to cause difficult milking. Warts on the udder are usually somewhat larger and more flattened than those on other parts of the skin (Fig. 7-2). As they are usually hard and dry in consistency, they are fairly easily removed. Frequently, warts spread from the original site to cover large areas of the body, either in the form of numerous

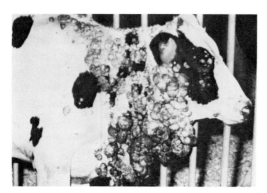

Fig. 7–1. Warts on neck of heifer.

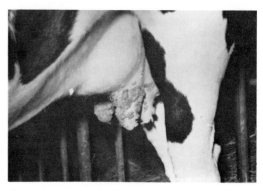

Fig. 7–2. Warts on udder of heifer.

nodules or as large confluent masses that may be either hard or soft in consistency. The soft masses bleed easily, have a tendency to slough, and give off an offensive odor. Upon autopsy, warts have also been found in the nasal openings of animals in the same herd. The agent apparently is transmitted by the fingers of a person who holds the animal or by an infected bull lead used as a means of restraint. The losses from warts are considerable. In young animals that are heavily infected with large warts, growth may be retarded. Greatest losses are the result of damages to the hides of slaughtered animals, brought about by the destruction of the hide where growth has occurred.

DIAGNOSIS

Diagnosis of infectious papillomatosis, or warts, is not difficult because the presence of dry, horny masses on the skin is significant. The warts affecting animals may clear up spontaneously with time. However, this time may be prolonged, and often curative treatment is needed. There are indications that recovered animals are resistant thereafter. Surgical removal of several large warts is often followed by dry necrosis of the stump and a spontaneous sloughing of the remaining warts.

TREATMENT

When a small number of warts appears on a single animal, or when a few animals in a group are affected, it may be advantageous for the herdsmen to tie off the warts with a sterile thread or string. When this procedure is done properly, the wart is constricted at its base, dry necrosis occurs, and the wart sloughs off; sloughing of all other warts on the body usually follows. Warts in cattle and goats sometimes respond to castor oil, acetic acid, or iodine applied locally before they become excessively enlarged.

If the condition is seen on a number of animals, or if an excessively large number of warts occurs on one animal, it may be advantageous to seek the advice of a veterinarian concerning a program of vaccination to insure that other susceptible animals on the premises do not become infected. Wart vaccines are available from commercial sources. They are made either from wart tissue treated with formalin and suspended in physiologic saline or from viruses isolated from such tissue and grown on chick embryo tissue culture. Wart tissue of bovine origin probably offers the most reliable vaccine source. These vaccines are given subcutaneously for prevention and treatment. The administration may be repeated at 5- to 10-day intervals, if necessary, but should be given only on the advice of a veterinarian.

Because the number of viruses actually involved in this particular condition is unknown, some commercial vaccines have proved ineffective. In such instances, successful results have been obtained by subsequent treatment with autogenous vaccine made from tissues taken from the specific herd. These results suggest that there may be immunologically different strains of a particular species.

Wart vaccine is administered subcutaneously or intracutaneously. It is claimed that a single injection leads to rapid regression of warts in some animals. Papillomas on the udder and teats do not respond as well to vaccine therapy as do those on other parts of the body.

The viruses causing infectious papillomatosis appear to have a high degree of host specificity, and some viruses even have specificities for particular kinds of epithelium within a single host. Although the viruses are host specific, all varieties are more prevalent within the young of the species affected.

For treating valuable herds that do not respond to other treatment, autogenous vaccine that is made from warty tissue taken from affected animals is recommended. Because it is prepared for individuals or a herd, autogenous vaccine should be used only in the herd from which it was collected.

PREVENTION

Once infectious papillomatosis has been diagnosed, severely infected animals should be isolated so that they do not come into contact with susceptible animals.

Barns, pens, chutes, and rubbing posts that infected cattle may have touched should be thoroughly cleaned. Remove manure, burn contaminated bedding and rubbish, and sweep and clean all free surfaces. Be particularly careful to remove cobwebs, dust, and other debris before washing the area with hot water and lye.

Once the area has been cleaned of all extraneous material and allowed to stand for a period of time, disinfect it by spraying a second time with the lye-and-water solution. Milk cows with warts on their teats and udders should be milked after all others in the herd have been milked. Clean and disinfect the milking machine teat cups and inflations before reusing. When cows are milked by hand during the treatment period, milkers should take stringent precautions to clean their hands with strong soap before milking other cows. In this way, there is less mechanical transmission from cow to cow.

Pinkeye

Pinkeye is an acute infectious disease of cattle, sheep, and, sometimes, other animals that is characterized by marked inflammation of the tissues of the eye and often designated by the synonyms *infectious bovine keratitis* and *infectious conjunctivitis*. It has been recognized since 1889 and is believed to be caused by a bacterium, Moraxella bovis, and an unclassified virus. The disease is widespread throughout the United States, especially among range and feedlot cattle. It is encountered in nearly half of all beef cattle herds and affects about 3% of all beef cattle.

Pinkeye occurs throughout the world and may appear in all seasons. It is most commonly seen in summer months, although there are reports of its occurrence during colder months, especially when the ground is covered with snow. It is always more prevalent when cattle are on the range without protection from intense light and especially during the seasons when flies are most active. Pinkeye affects animals of all ages, but animals under 2 years of age seem to be most susceptible.

Sheep and goats may also be affected, but this should not be confused with virus pinkeye. The bacterium Colesiota conjunctivae is the usual cause of pinkeye in sheep.

The severity of the disease and its yearly drain on the cattle industry are of great economic importance.

CAUSE

The disease has a complicated and unsettled cause. It is generally believed to be caused by Moraxella bovis and by a virus, either of which may act separately; both organisms are found in discharges from the eyes and noses of infected animals in which the primary lesions are confined to the cornea and conjunctiva. Some investigators have indicated that the Moraxella microorganism is the cause of infectious keratitis of cattle, but others believe that this cause has not definitely been established even though the microorganism is usually present in acute cases. Inability to agree on the role of M. bovis in pinkeye may be due to lack of uniformity in the types studied. It is possible that the differences may be accounted for by bacterial variation. M. bovis is a short, plump rod that usually occurs in pairs and short chains and is nonmotile, aerobic, gram-negative, and killed at 140°F in 5 minutes. Other bacteria are frequently isolated from infected cattle, and they are streptococci and staphylococci species. Both M. bovis and the virus have been studied separately and in pure form. Both have the ability to produce ocular lesions.

FACTORS INFLUENCING SUSCEPTIBILITY

Cattle of all ages and both sexes are susceptible, but pinkeye is more severe and frequent in those under 2 years of age. Dust, wind, bright sunlight, insects (especially flies), poor nutrition, vitamin A deficiency, and other conditions causing injury to the eye are usually predisposing causes. Cattle with nonpigmented faces, such as Herefords and Shorthorns, are severely affected.

TRANSMISSION

Cattle recovered from the disease might be able to spread the infection for several months after all symptoms have disappeared. Once the outbreak has started, microorganisms are rapidly spread by flies that cluster alternately around the eyes of infected and healthy animals. The disease is believed to be carried through the winter in a chronic form by carrier animals and seems to spread slightly before the arrival of flies. Secretions from the eyes have been demonstrated to contain M. bovis several months after an apparently complete recovery. Pinkeye may also be transmitted by direct contact and possibly by infected dust. Because nasal secretions of infected animals contain the causative agents, aerosols may be sprayed by coughing and sneezing. Common water troughs and feeding equipment also provide opportunities for spread of the disease. Introduction of carrier animals into susceptible

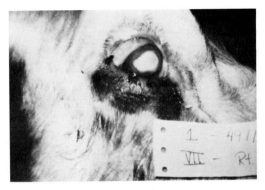

Fig. 7–3. Pinkeye with corneal opacity.

herds is a frequent method of initiating the disease within a herd.

CLINICAL SIGNS

Pinkeye is characterized by inflammation of the cornea, which is accompanied by nasal discharge, lacrimation, and copious ocular discharge that streams down the cheeks. The cornea turns a cloudy, opaque white, and eventually the eyelids close (Figs. 7-3, 7-4). In this condition, animals display extreme discomfort, and a sharp drop in milk production results. Affected animals behave as "loners," suffer injuries because of temporary blindness, and require special handling. In extreme

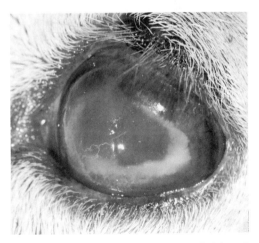

Fig. 7–4. Corneal opacity characteristic of pinkeye in cattle. (From Jensen, R, and Mackey, DR: Diseases of Feedlot Cattle. 2nd Edition. Philadelphia, Lea & Febiger, 1971.)

cases, permanent blindness occurs, greatly decreasing the value of the animal.

The incubation period is 3 to 5 days, and the average outbreak lasts about 3 weeks. Young animals are most seriously affected, and some older animals seem to retain considerable resistance after one attack, although they are not completely immune. Ulcers may form in severe instances on the front of one or both eyes near the pupil, and if progress is unchecked, they may cause blindness and even loss of the eye. The attack may also be marked by slight digestive upset. Most animals completely recover from the disease.

PATHOGENESIS

Rapid passage of the microorganism causing pinkeye through a succession of susceptible animals causes an increase in virulence. Once the causative agents localize in the eye, they cause injury to the epithelial cells of the conjunctiva and bring about circulatory disturbances accompanied by swelling and congestion. The cornea becomes edematous, with thickening, clouding, and opacity. Within a few days small ulcers form on the cornea; these may regress or coalesce to form larger ulcers and may penetrate into the deeper layers, resulting in loss of aqueous humor and lens. If regression does not occur, secondary pathogens gain entry through the cornea. In most animals, however, the infection is controlled before perforation of the cornea occurs, and the eye heals rapidly, usually with a residual scar of varying opacity.

DIAGNOSIS

Diagnosis is usually based on the appearance of the lesions. The disease may sometimes be confused with irritations caused by dust and wind, foreign bodies in the eye, or injuries by weed stems; however, there is of course no spreading from the latter conditions.

The disease may also be confused with the conjunctivitis caused by IBR and BVD. The distinction cannot be made merely by determining which comes first—the lesion on the cornea or the conjunctivitis. In fact, the IBR virus with M. bovis has been designated as causing outbreaks of pinkeye. The occular form of IBR must be ruled out before the diagnosis of pinkeye can be made. This can be done by serology or fluorescent antibody tests of conjunctival cells.

PREVENTION

Prevention can be based on eliminating the factors that predispose an animal to infection, such as dust, sunlight, and flies. Dust and sunlight certainly cannot be easily controlled, but efforts can be made to reduce spread by flies. Dusting or use of fly-repellent sprays gives temporary respite. Ear tags containing fly repellent have been effective. The incidence in white-face cattle has been reduced by painting dark rings around the eyes to reduce the effect of sunlight. Immunization with commercial vaccines has not been highly successful. Isolation or separation of infected cattle from those not showing signs of the disease may be of value if the disease has not already spread to apparently normal cattle.

If the condition cannot be distinguished from IBR or if the ocular form of IBR cannot be ruled out, the herd should be immunized against IBR.

TREATMENT

Treatment is difficult to evaluate because the condition spontaneously heals in many animals. Consequently, many different remedies are given credit for effecting a cure. Preparations of liquids or powders containing antibiotics or antibacterial properties have been extensively used by instilling in the eye. Eye ointments have been used. Because of the irritation of the medication, there is little residual effect as a result of lacrimation. A small amount of antibiotic injected into the conjunctiva to provide residual effect has become common practice. All methods have been evaluated, and results are not conclusive as to their efficacy.

Removing affected animals from environmental irritants by putting them in shaded, dust-free areas devoid of flies certainly enhances chances for healing. To give the eye the same type of protection, some cover the eye with a dark patch or sew the lids closed.

Contagious Ecthyma

Contagious ecthyma (sore mouth) is a contagious disease specific for sheep and goats. It is caused by a filterable virus and is characterized by the formation of papules, vesicles, pustules, and scabs on the lips, nose, muzzle, udder, and legs of sheep and goats. This disease is encountered in all parts of the world where sheep and goats are raised. The clinical signs are seen in late summer and fall in animals still on pasture, but later in the year in feedlots. The disease occurs most commonly in very young lambs in the spring, but rarely in mature sheep unless they have not been exposed to the virus in a previous season.

Historically, the disease was first described in Germany in the early 1920s. It was reported in Texas in 1929 and subsequently in all states where sheep and goats are raised. A successful vaccination was first reported in 1931.

CAUSE

Contagious ecthyma is caused by a single strain of a virus that is universal in distribution. The causative virus is present in the scabs removed from lesions on the skin of sheep and goats. It is resistant to desiccation and may be found in dried scabs in a protected area many years after the scabs have fallen from an infected lesion. One attack of the virus develops immunity in sheep. Lesions caused by the virus are susceptible to secondary invaders, such as bacteria or fly larvae.

TRANSMISSION

The virus is transmitted by direct contact between lambs and kids and by contact with contaminated feed and water. Young animals may become infected by nursing on dams with infected udders. Ewes and does themselves may develop lesions on the udder by nursing infected young. In very young lambs, the initial lesion may develop on the gum line below the incisor teeth. The native infection occurs by direct transfer of the virus into the tissues by means of slight wounds. Grass seed, spear grass, or other prickly plants that cause small puncture wounds or abrasions are the means by which the virus is spread from animal to animal. The virus cannot enter the tissues unless an abrasion or other type of injury provides a portal into the mucous membranes or skin.

FACTORS INFLUENCING SUSCEPTIBILITY

Sheep and goats are susceptible, but no other ruminants have been shown to be affected by the virus causing contagious ecthyma.

Young lambs and kids are most susceptible to the virus of contagious ecthyma, but older sheep not previously infected may have the disease in a mild form. Sheep of any age are susceptible unless they have been previously infected; however, once a sheep or goat has experienced the disease, a lasting immunity is developed. In areas of mild winter weather, the disease usually strikes in the early spring months and continues until cold weather begins. In the higher parts of the country, however, lambs are not usually infected until they are brought in from summer range. In some areas, husbandry methods at times of castrating and docking may lead to the production of the pox-like lesions through contaminating the mouth and gums of young lambs by careless handling.

CLINICAL SIGNS

The first sign is a slight swelling of the lips, followed by the appearance of small pustules that may break and exude pus. When these pustules dry, they form scabs that are yellowish-brown in color and may continue to thicken for a number of days. In approximately 3 weeks the scabs detach themselves and fall to the ground. The virus in the scabs remains viable for a considerable length of time, especially if protected from direct sunlight and chemical disinfectants. The laceration occurring beneath the scab and on the membranes on the inside of the mouth may serve as a focus for secondary invaders. In some animals, the legs may be affected. When the inflammation spreads to the tissues between the claws of the hoof, severe lameness occurs. Lesions may also occur on the anus, vulva, and udder of infected ewes.

The incubation period of the disease is from 2 to 8 days, and many lambs exhibit extremely sore and swollen dental pads and lips. No other signs are noted in uncomplicated cases, except extreme thinness caused by lack of food. Because of the soreness of the lips and tongue, newborn animals fail to nurse and thus predispose themselves to any other stress factor that may be present.

Secondary infections on the legs and feet may cause serious suppurative wounds that often spread up the leg.

Sometimes lesions are seen on other wool-free parts of the body; reddish, raised, spongy areas occur in the mouth, the gums, the dental pads, and palate. Removal of the scabs leaves a raw, inflamed, bleeding surface. Young animals may find suckling difficult, as the lips are immobile in badly affected cases and the animals may be in profound misery. Other complications may follow, producing separate sets of signs.

POSTMORTEM SIGNS

Upon postmortem examination, lesions are primarily found confined to the mouth parts or areas of the skin not covered by wool, but in cases of a secondary infection, one may observe ulcerative stomatitis, reticulitis, enteritis, necrotic pleural lesions with pleuritis, or necrotic foci in the liver. In some instances, the necrotic stomatitis may be extensive enough to cause a serious change in the shape or appearance of the lips of infected lambs. The disease produces typical lesions, but it may be confused with skin sensitization caused by other entities, such as mycotic dermatitis, photosensitivity, and poisoning or necrosis caused by heavy metal poisons.

TREATMENT

None of the current treatments is of any significance in preventing contagious ecthyma, and because the disease runs a benign course, treatment should not be attempted unless exceptional complications occur. In such instances, a veterinarian should be contacted to provide the latest information about treatments.

CONTROL

The control of contagious ecthyma takes two directions: (1) the immediate isolation of infected animals and the cleaning of contaminated areas, and (2) immunization.

Vaccination is quite effective. A vaccine made from the dried scabs of infected animals, diluted to a known strength, is used to vaccinate susceptible animals. However, a vaccine should not be used on premises where infection has never existed. Once the disease has appeared on a property, all susceptible animals must be vaccinated every year, as the virus has been known to live for as long as 12 years in scabs removed from infected animals. Vaccination can be carried out at any time, but it is usually done when lambs are gathered for docking. The vaccine is usually applied to skin in a wool-free area. A successful immunization is indicated by a reddened area a few days after scarification, followed by a pustule and a scab. Because the infection is spread predominantly at lambing time, all ordinary preventive precautions should be used at this time and sus-ceptible animals should be vaccinated to prevent the spread of the disease.

Public Health Relationships

Although the disease known as contagious ecthyma is rare in human beings, it can occur through careless handling of lambs and sheep. Gloves should be worn when vaccinating lambs, as vaccinating accidents do occur. In human infection, a papule develops, followed by a scab formation that heals in about 3 weeks unless complications occur. In some instances, especially when a human is bitten by a lamb suffering from this condition, lesions may develop on the hands and arms and regional lymph nodes may be involved. When this condition occurs, the healing process is protracted.

Vesicular Stomatitis

Vesicular stomatitis is a viral disease of cattle, swine, and, sometimes, horses and is characterized by inflammation of the tongue, the mucosa of the mouth, the coronary band of the hoof, and the formation of thin-walled vesicles containing clear or yellowish serous fluid. The disease may be transmitted to human beings. Public-health significance is related to the development of a systemic reaction and of mouth lesions among susceptible laboratory personnel, veterinarians, and farmers when exposed to the virus.

Geographically, vesicular stomatitis is considered to be confined to the western hemisphere. However, during periods of great movement of cattle and horses, the disease has spread to Europe; its current significance in Europe is unknown. Within the United States, vesicular stomatitis is primarily found in the southeastern part of the United States, although it has spread in the past through the cattle-raising areas of the middle west. Because it is prevalent where the climate is temperate, the disease is endemic in some areas in the United States at all times during the year.

Historically, the disease was first described in horses during World War I and subsequently in horses shipped to Europe during that period of time. It was first described in cattle in 1926 and in swine in 1943.

CAUSE

Vesicular stomatitis is caused by a virus. The host range includes sheep, dogs, deer, bobcats, many rodents, and cold-blooded animals. The virus may be propagated in tissue culture in the laboratory and on chicken embryos. However, because vesicular stomatitis in cattle and swine is clinically indistinguishable from foot-and-mouth disease and vesicular exanthema, a differential diagnosis is of great importance.

Two types of the virus are described in the United States: the Indiana type and the

New Jersey type. Each of these is immunologically different from the other; however, the New Jersey type is considered more prevalent and possibly more virulent than the Indiana type. The virus, found in abundance in the clear, vesicular fluid and the vesicular covering, is most infective when the vesicles rupture or shortly thereafter. It may be found in the blood during the febrile stage of the disease and for a short period afterward. However, once the blisters or vesicles have burst, the virus can no longer be recovered from the blood.

The virus remains active for several days at body temperatures, but is rapidly killed by direct sunlight. It is also susceptible to solutions of formalin, cresylic-acid soaps, and hypochlorite, as is foot-and-mouth disease virus.

TRANSMISSION

Transmission of vesicular stomatitis virus is by direct contact with the saliva or material contaminated by the saliva of infected animals, and by the vesicular fluid expressed from ruptured vesicles. Mechanical transmission by insects has been demonstrated in the laboratory, and because infections usually vanish with the first frost, insect vectors have been incriminated as a means of transmission of the virus. Abrasions of the mouth, feet, or teats facilitate successful establishment and growth of the virus found on feed materials. Crowding of animals tends to lead to a spread of vesicular stomatitis; however, the disease is seen more frequently among animals on pasture than in those crowded into feedlots.

FACTORS INFLUENCING SUSCEPTIBILITY

The incidence of vesicular stomatitis in all livestock appears to be greater during the warm summer than during the winter. Infection ceases with the first frost, lending credence to the assumption that an insect vector is the source of spread and the reservoir over the winter months. Age appears to be associated with susceptibility in cattle, as the disease rarely appears in cattle less than 1 year of age. However, in swine, the disease occurs in suckling pigs as well as in older animals. There appears to be no age susceptibility influence in horses.

Feeding on plants with acrid substance on the leaves (clover, rape, and similar roughages) may produce slight irritation or abrasions in the mouth; these facilitate the entrance of viruses that may be on the pasture plants or in feed material or drinking troughs.

CLINICAL SIGNS

The incubation period for the virus appears to be 2 to 5 days, during which the temperature may rise to 105°F; however, once the vesicles have formed and ruptured, the temperature decreases rapidly. The first signs noted in dairy cattle are a loss of milk secretion and a beginning of loss of condition. Examination of the animal at this time reveals lesions in the mouth varying from very small to pea size. When a small vesicle ruptures, others may rapidly develop around the site and coalesce to involve a considerable portion or the entire surface of the tongue or lips. These lesions cause pain, resulting in loss of appetite, lowered milk secretion, and loss of condition. The lesions may cover the entire surface of the teats or may occur as isolated vesicles on one or more teats. Lesions may also appear in the interdigital spaces between the claws, but are usually confined to only one foot. In swine, the vesicular lesions may appear on the snout and on the coronary band around the foot. Lesions on teats and feet do not occur as frequently as in other vesicular diseases. In the average herd afflicted with vesicular stomatitis, the morbidity rate is approximately 50%; however, if blood samples are taken for laboratory diagnosis, 100% of the animals in the herd may show antibodies indicative of a frank or inapparent infection.

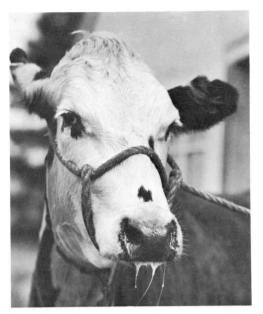

Fig. 7–5. Typical appearance of vesicular stomatitis in a cow 48 hours after experimental inoculation with the virus.

The lesions appearing on the mouth, tongue, gums, lips, and even extending to the nostrils on cattle and swine appear first as small macules, or raised pimples, which develop quickly into full-blown vesicles. The vesicles are filled with a straw-colored clear fluid in which the virus propagates rapidly and which may serve as a source of contamination for other animals (Fig. 7-5). Once the vesicles rupture, the site heals quickly; however, there may be time for entry of secondary invaders, causing additional ulceration and pain. Vesicles on the tongue usually rupture and leave a denuded area that may be extensive (Fig. 7-6), sometimes including the entire epithelium of the upper surface, with bluish discoloration; this can lead to secondary bacterial invasion.

PATHOGENESIS

The virus gains entry through abrasions in the mouth, around the coronary band of the hoof, or on the teat surfaces. Production of macules, vesicles, and erosions follows the rupture of the vesicles. After invasion, the virus enters the lower level of the skin, attacks epithelial cells, and grows rapidly. In a few hours, many cells are injured and the viral particles are released; the virus then invades other cells closer to the surface of the skin, and the resulting vesicles are formed. The virus appears in the blood during this stage of the disease, but the infective stage decreases after the vesicles have ruptured. Within 3 to 4 days, the virus can no longer be demonstrated in either the blood or the saliva.

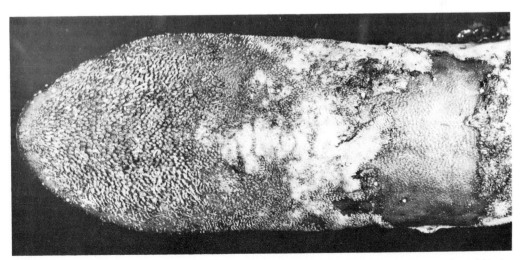

Fig. 7–6. Bovine tongue showing denuded area resulting from vesicular stomatitis. (From Jensen, R, and Mackey, DR: Diseases of Feedlot Cattle. 2nd Edition. Philadelphia, Lea & Febiger, 1971.)

DIAGNOSIS

The clinical diagnosis of vesicular stomatitis is based on the occurrence of typical oral, foot, or mammary lesions in adult cattle and swine during warm months in a known enzootic area. Because of the similarity of this disease to foot-and-mouth disease and vesicular exanthema, great care must be exercised in arriving at a positive diagnosis. Whenever there is a question, expert veterinary assistance and laboratory confirmation must be obtained.

TREATMENT

In the past, commercial vaccines have been available to combat this disease on a herd basis. However, because the disease is reportable in most states and because eradication methods have been successful, vaccines are no longer necessary. Should an outbreak occur, vaccines to combat the ravages of the disease in endemic areas could be readily obtained.

PREVENTION

Prevention is based primarily on good management procedures, that is, a strict quarantine and the banning of shipment of animals for a minimum of 30 days after all evidence of an infection has passed. Recovered animals are immune for 2 to 3 months; however, no cross immunity exists with other vesicular diseases or from one type of vesicular stomatitis virus to another type. Thus, all infected animals must be segregated and separate feeding equipment and material must be used when the disease has been diagnosed. Even though strict quarantine is seldom applied, owners of diseased cattle should avoid direct or indirect exposure of other feedlots or farms. Flying and crawling insects should be controlled and palliative treatment of the complicated vesicles should be initiated.

CHAPTER 8
Exotic Diseases

This chapter includes brief descriptions of several diseases currently not found in North America. Their presence in other areas is a constant threat to the livestock industry. The possibility of delayed diagnosis because of the similarity of their signs to signs of other diseases, e.g., hog cholera and African swine fever, BVD and rinderpest, foot-and-mouth and other vesicular diseases, is reason to take immediate steps to investigate the slightest suspicion of their presence. The Animal and Plant Health Inspection Service of the USDA must be notified to provide diagnostic confirmation (see Chap. 1, Agencies of Disease Control).

RECOMMENDED READING

Dunne, HW, and Leman, AD: Diseases of Swine. 4th Edition. Chap. 9. Ames, IA, Iowa State University Press, 1975.

Committee on Foreign Animal Diseases of the United States Animal Health Association: African Swine Fever. *In* Foreign Animal Diseases: Their Prevention, Diagnosis, and Control. 3rd Edition. Washington, Government Printing Office, 1975, pp. 43-53.

————: Rinderpest. *In* Foreign Animal Diseases: Their Prevention, Diagnosis, and Control. 3rd Edition. Washington, Government Printing Office, 1975, pp. 222-233.

————: African Horse Sickness. *In* Foreign Animal Diseases: Their Prevention, Diagnosis, and Control. 3rd Edition. Washington, Government Printing Office, 1975, pp. 31-41.

African Swine Fever

African swine fever is a highly contagious peracute disease of domestic swine. It is characterized by fever; pronounced hemorrhages of the lymphatic glands, kidneys, and mucosa of the alimentary tract; marked cyanosis of areas on the skin; and mortality approaching 100%. Clinically, African swine fever resembles acute hog cholera, but it is an immunologically distinct entity. It is the most deadly of all foreign diseases of swine.

CAUSE AND DISTRIBUTION

The causal agent is an exceptionally resistant filterable virus. Infective blood stored at ordinary room temperature may remain virulent after 18 months and, when stored in a cold room (4 to 5°C), can still be active after 6 years. The bush pig and warthog can harbor the virus, but usually show no objective symptoms. Viremia is a consistent feature of this disease, and all tissues, organs, and excreta contain the virus.

In South Africa, outbreaks of swine fever were recorded from 1903 to 1935. In East Africa, in areas where contact with other domestic pigs could be definitely excluded, it was determined that the African virus differed from the virus of classic hog cholera. Wild pigs were incriminated as inapparent carriers from which domestic pigs obtained the infection. Researchers were also able to infect susceptible pigs by inoculating them with blood collected from a number of apparently healthy warthogs. However, blood obtained from warthogs in other areas proved to be non-infective.

Prior to 1957, African swine fever was confined to continental Africa. In that year, the disease appeared in Portugal, and in 1964, it appeared in France. By 1967, the disease had spread to Italy, causing a serious threat to swine in the rest of Europe and other swine-raising areas of the world.

In May of 1971, the disease was diagnosed for the first time in the western hemisphere, in Cuba. By quarantine and eventual slaughter of over 400,000 hogs, control was established in August, 1971.

In March, 1981, the USDA declared an animal health emergency because of an outbreak of African swine fever in Haiti. The proximity of Haiti to the United States posed a threat to the U.S. swine industry. A cooperative effort with the government of Haiti has been planned to prevent spread of the disease and to eradicate it in Haiti.

TRANSMISSION

Wild boars or bush pigs and warthogs serve as reservoirs of the disease in Africa. Contact of domestic swine with wild pigs harboring the virus may initiate the disease. Once the disease is established in domestic swine, it spreads rapidly by contact.

Urine and feces from infected hogs contain the virus in sufficient amounts to infect susceptible hogs. The virus can be spread mechanically by caretakers and others who pass from infected premises without taking proper measures of disinfection. Meat from infected animals contains the virus, and as with hog cholera, the feeding of raw garbage may spread the disease. In South Africa, infected pigs were deliberately slaughtered and their carcasses were sent to bacon factories; this bacon was the source of sporadic outbreaks of disease for some considerable period. Attempts to transmit this disease by lice and fleas have been inconsistent, although Spanish scientists have found that it may be transmitted by a tick.

In a few instances in which swine have survived this disease, there is evidence that they may act as carriers for as long as 10 months after recovery. Investigators have failed to demonstrate that contact of susceptible hogs with warthogs with blood harboring the virus resulted in infection of the hogs. For this reason, the theory has been advanced that infection may be transmitted from warthogs to pigs by an insect vector or by pigs actually eating carcasses of virus-carrying wild pigs.

CLINICAL SIGNS

Unless the herd is under close observation, the first indication of the disease may be the discovery of one or two dead pigs. On close observation, the first sign is a marked rise in temperature to 104 to 108° F. About 24 hours prior to death, sick animals become dull and listless, refuse to eat, and may be found lying huddled in a corner and disinclined to move. When forced to rise, they exhibit a swaying movement and weakness of the hindquarters. The hindquarter weakness is less prevalent and less severe in African swine fever than in American hog cholera. Cyanosis of the skin on the ears, snout, abdomen, and legs is usually pronounced. In about 40% of the cases, pulmonary involvement is sufficient to cause labored respiration. Associated heart rate is accelerated to 180 beats per minute and is irregular. Pregnant sows usually abort. Some strains may produce a mucopurulent discharge from the eyes and a mucous discharge from the nostrils. Constipation is frequently present, although diarrhea, usually bloody, may develop. Death generally occurs on the fourth to seventh day after the onset of signs and is preceded by a marked drop in temperature. For about 24 hours before death, an infected animal is comatose, lying on its side with stretched-out legs and closed eyes and grunting only feebly when stirred. The disease is so highly contagious that, in a few days after the first incidence is noticed, most swine in the herd have become infected and have a rise of temperature. Nevertheless, in Africa, the virus from the warthog or wild pig frequently appears to take some time to attain high virulence. Thus, a common history of outbreak is an isolated death that is followed a week or so later by one or two more deaths, and then, after a further interval, by many cases with rapid spread.

The incubation period is usually 4 to 7 days when exposure is by contact with infected pigs.

POSTMORTEM SIGNS

The outstanding lesions are hemorrhages, thrombosis, infarction, hyalinization, and necrosis of the internal organs. These changes are caused by damage done by the virus to the endothelial cells of the small blood vessels, for which it seems to have a predilection.

The skin almost invariably has a patchy or diffuse purplish color and, more rarely, single or multiple irregular, dark red, hemorrhagic patches distributed on the abdomen, head, and limbs.

On opening the carcass, one may be startled by the degree of hemorrhage seen. The internal lymph glands may be deep bluish-black because of extravasation of blood into the reticular spaces and lymph sinuses. The hemorrhage is often so extensive that the glands appear as blood clots. The lungs may be cyanotic and, in some instances, edemic; they are often dark and swollen to as much as twice the normal size. Engorgement of the blood vessels of the gallbladder is common.

Hyperemia, severe enough to cause hemorrhage, is fairly consistent in the mucosa of the stomach.

The stomach is usually full of food. The changes in the small intestine vary from no change to severe hyperemia with hemorrhagic or even diphtheritic enteritis. There is often marked edema in the walls of the cecum, spiral colon, and the mesentery of these organs, thus giving a gelatinous appearance. A hemorrhagic inflammation of the rectum is characteristic. However, the lesions encountered in African swine fever may vary considerably, and animals may die of this disease without showing any obvious gross lesions.

DIAGNOSIS

In Africa, a diagnosis can be made when characteristic symptoms and lesions occur in swine that have had possible contact with wild pigs.

African swine fever so closely resembles hog cholera that a clinical or pathologic differentiation is difficult to make. A presumptive diagnosis can be based on gross postmortem signs—the marked severity of the lesions of African swine fever, especially the hemorrhagic lymph glands and vascular engorgement of the mesentery,

and particularly in swine that have been vaccinated against hog cholera.

The conclusive method of diagnosis is the production of the disease, under strict isolation, by inoculating susceptible swine (including cholera-immune and hyperimmunized pigs) with suspect material, such as blood or spleen taken from a recently dead animal. Swine that are immune and even hyperimmune to hog cholera are susceptible to African swine fever, and this fact is of value in making a differential diagnosis. Laboratory tests are available but time consuming.

CONTROL

African swine fever is undoubtedly the most serious of the exotic diseases insofar as the swine industries of the United States and Canada are concerned.

The best available methods of control are to slaughter all infected and exposed animals immediately, to dispose of all carcasses by burning or deep burial, to disinfect the infected premises, and to quarantine infected areas. In Africa, measures taken to prevent contact of domestic swine with wild pigs have resulted in a marked decrease in incidence of the disease.

Although work to produce a vaccine continues, immunization is not an effective control measure for this disease at present.

Rinderpest

Rinderpest, or cattle plague, is an acute, highly contagious, generalized viral disease, primarily of cattle and secondarily of sheep, goats, and wild ruminants. The disease is characterized by a rapidly fatal, febrile course with inflammation and necrosis of the mucous membranes of the digestive tract leading to emaciation and profuse bloody diarrhea. Rinderpest infects wild and domesticated pigs; horses,

carnivorous animals, and man are not susceptible.

Since ancient times, rinderpest has been the world's most devastating disease of cattle, and as such, it has had a major influence on man's food supply. In many parts of the world, cattle plagues were devastating from the fifth century until development of methods of disease control in the present century. It has been estimated that, before 1949, rinderpest was responsible for the loss of more than 2 million cattle and buffalo each year, and it is only through modern prophylactic measures, persistently pursued, that large-scale raising of cattle has today become profitable in much of Africa and in the Middle East and Asia.

There are numerous mentions in the literature of scourges of rinderpest that wiped out cattle in many parts of the civilized world following military campaigns of the past. More recently, commercial shipments of live animals from one part of the world to another have introduced rinderpest into many countries that were formerly free of the disease. It is not present in the western hemisphere or in western Europe only because stringent methods have been exercised to keep it out. In fact, one outbreak did occur in Brazil in 1921, but prompt methods of eradication were exercised, and rinderpest has not appeared again in this part of the world. However, it is still enzootic in most of Africa, Asia, and the Middle East. In tropical Africa, it occurs in different degrees of severity. In eastern Europe, outbreaks continue to occur periodically, although the disease has not been diagnosed in western Europe since 1920.

The persistent use of modern vaccines and drastic tests and slaughter procedures have eradicated rinderpest from the Philippine Islands, Australia, New Zealand, and Japan.

CAUSE

Rinderpest is caused by a relatively fragile virus ranging in size from 120 to 300 mμ. Although all field strains of virus have been reported as immunologically similar, they vary widely in pathogenicity, lethality, ease of transmission, and host affinity. Prolonged passage of the virus in cattle may cause it to lose its capacity for natural transmission. Serial passage of some strains of the virus in goats, rabbits, chick embryos, and tissue cultures has lead to attenuation for cattle. Some of these attenuated strains have been widely used in vaccines. There also appears to be an immunologic relationship between rinderpest virus and the viruses of measles and canine distemper. Because of the fragile nature of the virus, it loses its infectiveness within a matter of hours in a moist medium at room temperature; it does, however, remain infectious for many days under refrigeration. When the virus is frozen, it remains infectious for a considerable length of time. Strong alkalis, acids, and the common disinfectants destroy the virus.

In the infected animals, however the virus is extremely virulent and may be found in large quantities in blood, tissue fluids, secretions, and excretions; it is also present in meat from slaughtered animals.

FACTORS INFLUENCING SUSCEPTIBILITY

In enzootic areas where most mature cattle acquire some degree of immunity, many cases of rinderpest are mild and inapparent. Because of this degree of resistance or immunity acquired through generations of exposure in enzootic areas, the disease is most often seen in young animals. Sex is of no importance in the transmission or incidence of the disease, but good condition appears to make animals more resistant. There is no relationship of the disease to either season, climate, or weather. The appearance of rinderpest in sheep and goats is relatively rare, but there have been instances of the infection appearing in swine. Reports of outbreaks are rather common in certain native breeds of swine in the Far East. The disease, however, has not been reported among African wild swine or hogs. In enzootic areas, native cattle (exposed to rinderpest for generations) are generally more resistant than newly imported breeds. Contrary to the rule, however, a few native breeds in enzootic areas have remained susceptible to the disease.

TRANSMISSION

Rinderpest is usually transmitted by direct contact between infected and susceptible ruminants, and the movement of infected animals is primarily responsible for the spread of the disease. The ingestion of virus-contaminated feed or water may transmit the disease, but based on experimental transmissions, the chances of transmission are much more likely to occur by way of the respiratory tract from the inhalation of virus-laden aerosols from infected animals. There is evidence that, on rare occasions, a recovered animal may continue to harbor and excrete the virus for several weeks after the first development of the disease; however, immune carriers are not considered to be a prevalent factor in transmission.

The major means of transmission has been considered to be droplet infection onto the conjunctiva, internal nares, and respiratory tract; however, it has been experimentally shown that infective material placed upon the external nares, lips, mouth, esophagus, and the first three stomachs rarely produces the disease.

The mechanical transmission of rinderpest by biting insects appears possible, but there is no evidence in the literature that insects are involved in the natural transmission of the disease. With some virulent strains of rinderpest, the virus may be disseminated by an infected animal 1 or 2 days before the animal shows signs of apparent illness. The dissemination of virus prior to apparent illness poses a major control problem for animals kept in congested sales yards or in transit. All tissues and excretions from infected animals should be considered infectious throughout the period of clinical illness.

CLINICAL SIGNS

In general, three forms of the disease may be described: (1) typically acute; (2) subacute, occurring primarily in countries where the disease is enzootic; and (3) peracute. Various atypical forms of the disease are sometimes seen. Many of the unusual features are the result of complications caused by concurrent or superimposed viral infections. Rinderpest can be so highly contagious that, when cattle infected with a virulent strain of bovine virus are allowed to mingle with susceptible cattle, the morbidity may approach 100%, and among highly susceptible cattle, mortality may reach 90%. Recovery confers a permanent immunity, and the development of immune carriers able to disperse the disease to susceptible cattle has not been reported. A temporary maternal immunity protects the calves of immune dams for the first several months of life. When this maternal immunity is present, it proportionately lessens the effectiveness of vaccination.

Although the method of transmission of the disease is direct, the rinderpest virus enters the body primarily through the digestive tract and passes to the blood where it propagates rapidly. It is transmitted then to the mucous membranes of the digestive tract, for which it seems to possess a degree of selectivity. In any case, the virus enters the capillary epithelium, causing an inflammatory process accompanied by early necrosis of epithelial cells; these cells erode, causing the serious bloody diarrhea that is one of the common signs of the disease. In natural outbreaks, the period of incubation varies from 3 to 9 days. In countries where the disease is enzootic, the incubation period may be somewhat longer. Artificial infection by inoculation results in a rather short incubation period of 40 to 60 hours.

Differences in strain virulence and in host susceptibility account for a wide range of clinical severity from inapparent to peracute cases. After natural infection and an incubation period of 3 to 15 days, the onset in cattle is typically marked by an abrupt rise in temperature to 104 to 105° F. Within 48 hours after the temperature rise, nasal and lacrimal discharges appear and are accompanied by depression, thirst, and loss of appetite. The pulse and respiration are accelerated, and milk secretion diminishes or ceases. The conjunctiva is deeply infected and copious lacrimation occurs. It has been reported that congestion of the vaginal mucosa usually precedes all other lesions. Similar lesions are found in the preputial mucosa of the male. On the second or third day of fever, small gray papules (about the size of a pinhead) are usually found in small numbers on the gums, lips, and undersurfaces of the tongue. During the next 24 hours, vesicles form in these papules and rupture to form ulcers; a fresh crop of papules then develops. These oral lesions apparently induce excessive salivation as they increase in severity. The saliva, however, does not form the long, tenacious, mucoid strings common in foot-and-mouth disease.

The temperature reaches its peak by the third to fifth day, and diarrhea commonly starts with the drop in temperature to normal or subnormal levels. As the diarrhea increases in severity, it may become hemorrhagic and is associated with abdominal pain, accelerated respiration, occasional cough, severe dehydration, and emaciation followed by prostration and death. The feces, which were at first dry and covered with mucus, become soft and finally blackish, liquid, and often blood-stained. There may be twitching of superficial muscles, grinding of teeth, and arching of the back. Animals show extreme depression with occasional periods of excitement. Animals often die in the second day of this phase; if not, diarrhea continues, and they become debilitated, remain recumbent, waste rapidly, and finally die, usually between 4 to 8 days after the first appearance of fever.

In some animals, the respiratory tract is affected. A nasal discharge develops, which later becomes purulent and blood-stained. There may be bronchial rales and coughing. Pregnant animals frequently abort.

In the *peracute* form of the disease, there is marked congestion of the mucosa and great acceleration of pulse and respiration. Death may occur before diarrhea develops. This form is common in calves, which may die on the second or third day without showing typical buccal lesions.

The *subacute* form occurs primarily in animals in countries where the disease is enzootic. The clinical features are essentially the same as those in the acute cases, although milder and more prolonged.

Atypical forms are sometimes seen. Cutaneous lesions may develop in the form of red maculae, either separate or confluent on various parts of the body and most often where the skin is thin. They pass through papular and vesicle pustular stages and may be followed by shedding of patches of epidermis.

In buffalo, camels, sheep, and goats, the clinical features vary from those seen in typical acute cases in cattle to those of a mild form that may not be fatal. In general, the disease in sheep and goats is much milder than in cattle. Swine, both domesticated and wild, show variable forms of the disease. Infection of adult hogs by ingestion or subcutaneous inoculation usually produces a hypothermia that lasts several days without the development of any striking signs of illness, although the blood is infective. Young swine appear to show severe clinical disease more frequently after inoculation, with lesions in the buccal cavity, mucopurulent conjunctivitis, and diarrhea.

POSTMORTEM SIGNS

Because the virus has a particular affinity for the epithelial linings of the digestive tract and lymphoid tissues, the predominant postmortem signs seen in cattle that have died of rinderpest are related to these tissues and structures. The animals commonly show the effect of the severe diarrhea. They are dehydrated and emaciated, and the hair coat is rough and soiled. Although, in rare instances, death may occur prior to the development of the characteristic lesions, necropsies conducted on several animals in an outbreak usually include the following changes.

The rinderpest virus has affinity for and is highly destructive to the lymphoid tissues. Grossly, the lymph nodes are soft, edematous, and moderately enlarged. Peyer's patches show the most marked gross evidence of lymphoid destruction. Located in an exposed area and composed of highly susceptible digestive tract mucosae and lymphoid tissue, they usually become acutely inflamed; later, necrosis and erosion may leave raw craters at the site of the patches.

The epithelial lining of the mouth and digestive tract is highly vulnerable to the rinderpest virus. The initial lesions in the oral epithelium include formation and necrosis of a few papular-like lesions. The extension of this necrosis toward the surface indicates an increase in the size of the necrotic lesions. The first such lesions to be grossly evident occur on the intersurfaces of the lower lip, adjacent to the gum, on the cheeks, and on the ventral surfaces of the tongue. Later, these erosions may enlarge and coalesce to involve most of the oral mucosa.

Gross lesions are only occasionally found in the rumen and reticulum, but hemorrhages and erosions appear fairly frequent in the omasum.

Extensive congestion and hemorrhage are associated with the degeneration, necrosis, and erosion of the mucosae of the abomasum and the intestines. Erosions here leave a raw, bleeding surface. Edema, hemorrhage, and erosions of the mucosa of the gastric fundus are often found. The small intestine usually shows slight involvement except for frequent necrosis and erosion of the Peyer's patches.

The most frequent lesions are seen in the large intestine and involve the cecum, the cecocolic junction, and the rectum. The upper respiratory passages may be congested, but most often, the nasal mucosa is markedly hyperemic, showing some hemorrhages and covered more or less uniformly with mucopurulent exudate, ac-companied by some ulceration. Similar lesions may also be found in the trachea. At the commencement of an outbreak, death may occur so rapidly that typical lesions are not apparent.

DIAGNOSIS

The diagnosis of rinderpest in countries where the disease is prevalent is based on clinical features, or gross lesions, and a knowledge of the history of the disease in a given area. The clinical and gross pathologic features of rinderpest, which are much like those seen in viral diarrhea and mucosal diseases, require that particular emphasis be placed on proper laboratory diagnosis when the disease is suspected to have occurred in a country normally free of rinderpest. A presumptive diagnosis must be confirmed by serologic means, utilizing neutralization tests either in cattle or in tissue culture, or by cross-protection tests in cattle. A knowledge of the disease is essential to facilitate prompt recognition.

CONTROL

Any regimen of control of rinderpest is based first on proper sanitation and elimination of the virus. Because of the failure of the virus to survive for any length of time outside the animal body, sanitation and disinfection facilitate control of the disease. Clean quarters that are well ventilated and exposed to sunlight and the proper application of thorough disinfection techniques help to prevent the spread of the disease.

In areas where the disease is common, immunization techniques have been used. When the disease is too widespread for the costly measures of slaughter and quarantine, control can be achieved through vaccination and isolation. Two types of vaccines are commonly used: (1) a killed virus, and (2) an attenuated virus that has been passed through unusual hosts. The current use of attenuated vaccines has largely outmoded older vaccines that used modified live viruses and killed viruses.

These attenuated vaccines are produced by serial passage through goats, rabbits, chick embryos, and also tissue cultures.

In the United States, the prevention of the entry of the disease is still the primary method of control, and should an outbreak occur, the drastic measures of tests, slaughter, and disposal would be undertaken. Rinderpest has been designated a reportable disease by all state and federal authorities, and the federal government has placed an embargo on the importation of cattle from countries where the disease is known to exist.

Foot-and-Mouth Disease

Foot-and-mouth disease, also known as aphthous fever and aftosa, is an acute, febrile, highly contagious disease of cloven-footed animals. It is caused by a filterable virus and is characterized by the formation of vesicles in the buccal mucous membrane, in the skin above the hoof, and in the interdigital spaces. The first recorded outbreak of this disease was in Europe in 1544. In 1897, European scientists determined the cause. These investigators showed that bacteria-free lymph collected from infected animals could be used to transmit the infection. Later, in 1898, they proved that the causative agent of foot-and-mouth disease could be passed through filters that retained bacteria.

Foot-and-mouth disease occurs in most of the cattle-raising regions of the world. The disease has never obtained a foothold in Australia, New Zealand, and North America because these regions have long used drastic means of prevention. There have been nine outbreaks in the United States, but each was successfully stamped out without excessive cost or extensive loss of cattle. The disease continues to be of great interest to animal disease-control authorities because of the great outbreak that occurred in Mexico between 1946 and 1954. In 1951 to 1952, a small outbreak in western Canada, close to the international border, caused considerable concern in this country. Most of the North American outbreaks have been traced to contaminated products imported from other countries.

CAUSE

The filterable virus causing foot-and-mouth disease is one of the smallest viruses known; it is about 22 mμ in diameter and spherical in shape. There are seven types of the virus and at least 61 subtypes, all of which are antigenically distinct. Three types have thus far been reported from Africa, whereas the others have been found in various parts of the world. Each of the seven types produces a disease picture comparable to the other six.

The virus appears to be quite sensitive to heat and is removed from milk through standard pasteurization. When kept in an incubator at about 98° F, the virus loses infectivity within 48 hours. At average room temperature, it remains viable for 2 to 3 weeks. At ordinary refrigeration temperatures, the virus usually remains infective for many months when properly buffered. When rapidly dried under vacuum at low temperatures, it remains viable for several years. The virus is more sensitive to acids than to alkalis and is resistant to alcohol, ether, chloroform, and other fat solvents. The cultivation of the virus is usually accomplished by the inoculation of scarified areas of the buccal mucosa and tongue of calves, by footpad inoculation of guinea pigs, and by tissue-culture techniques in the laboratory.

TRANSMISSION

Respiratory aerosols from infected animals and ingestion of contaminated food and water are the principal means of transmission of the disease. Although indirect transmission may take place by contact with inanimate objects of various kinds, the spread of foot-and-mouth disease is primarily by and from infected animals. The virus may also be transmitted from the surroundings of infected animals by people, horses, dogs, birds, flies, rats, and inanimate articles, such as harnesses, vehicles, brushes, and clothing that may be contaminated with saliva, urine, feces, milk, and meat of infected animals.

FACTORS INFLUENCING SUSCEPTIBILITY

Susceptibility to natural infection of this disease is almost exclusively limited to cloven-footed animals, both domestic and wild. Cattle, hogs, sheep, and goats are most frequently affected (in the order mentioned). Deer were seriously affected in an outbreak in California, and naturally infected hedgehogs have been found in England. The virus does not persist in animals in the carrier state with any regularity, but the disease has recurred on farms as long as a year following eradication procedures.

Carnivorous animals are resistant and solipeds are completely immune to this disease; however, dogs and cats, especially the young, are slightly susceptible to artificial infection. Young farm animals on a high level of nutrition are most easily and acutely infected. Purebred animals seem to be more susceptible than grade animals, and close housing and feeding are conducive to the spread of the disease. Debilitated animals frequently suffer more from secondary effects. The severity of the disease varies with the strain of the virus and the state of health of the herd.

CLINICAL SIGNS

The disease is characterized by depression, fever, and the appearance of vesicles filled with clear fluid in oral mucous membranes and portions of the skin. The virus multiplies only in the inner layers of epithelium, where it causes degenerative changes and separation of these layers from the more superficial cornified layer. This space then fills with fluid and thus forms vesicles. The vesicles generally appear on the mucous membranes of the mouth (tongue, cheeks, dental pad, and gums), on the skin of the muzzle, in the interdigital spaces, around the tops of the claws, on the teats and, occasionally, on the surface of the udder. Vesicles may also appear around the base of the horns and in the pharynx, larynx, trachea, esophagus, and wall of the rumen around the esophageal groove.

These pathologic changes in the tissues produce a series of other signs, such as an increase in body temperature, loss of appetite, lassitude, and profuse slobbering (Fig. 8-1). Because chewing may be painful, the animal may eat little or not at all and, therefore, loses condition and weight. Infected animals usually become lame, and milk flow usually ceases. Abortion, mastitis, and infertility may also occur. The incubation period following natural exposure is 2 to 7 days. Within 24 to 48

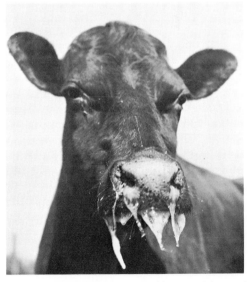

Fig. 8–1. Cow slobbering, an early sign of foot-and-mouth disease.

hours after multiplication of the virus in the epithelium, the virus escapes into the blood and is carried to all organs and tissues. This spread often results in the appearance of secondary vesicles in epithelium remote from the point of entry of the virus. Although the virus does not multiply in the blood or organs, it does produce degenerative changes in muscular tissues, particularly in the heart. Yellowish streaks and foci of parenchymatous degeneration are the manifestations of this damage.

PATHOGENESIS

The vesicles in the mouth, 0.5 to 10.0 centimeters in diameter and circular, rupture within a few hours of their formation, leaving large flaps of whitish, detached epithelium under which the tissues are raw and bleeding. Often, a large part of the tongue is denuded. Secondary bacterial infections of the denuded areas between the claws usually occur and result in deep necrosis of tissues and suppuration that frequently undermines the claws, causing them to be loosened from the soft tissues and eventually to be sloughed off. The mouth lesions usually heal within 1 to 3 days, but the foot lesions often persist much longer.

The virus reaches the epithelium in the region in which it localizes either by direct contact or by way of the blood. Two to seven days after the virus enters the epithelium, vesicles and erosions develop. The epithelial cells in the lesions begin to enlarge and undergo a liquefaction degeneration sometimes called hydropic degeneration. The intercellular bridges disappear, and the cells consequently become loosened from one another. Their nuclei become pyknotic. Separation of the epithelium is aided by the endematous fluid arising from the hyperemic vessels of the skin. Adjacent foci, thus filled with edema fluid arising from cells undergoing liquefaction degeneration, fuse to form small vesicles. Small vesicles coalesce to form larger vesicles. Internal pressure within the vesicles becomes great, and the superficial cover-

ing becomes increasingly thinner. This thinning, plus softening caused by excessive saliva, leads to rupture of vesicles.

Loss of epithelium is most common on the dorsal surface of the anterior part of the bovine tongue. The entire epithelium over the anterior area may be lost, leaving a raw, red surface that oozes blood. In addition to the virus, the vesicles contain necrotic epithelial cells, leukocytes, occasional erythrocytes and, in the late stages, bacteria. Lesions in the myocardium are most common in fatal cases of foot-and-mouth disease. The lesions, observed in the wall and septum of the left ventricle but seldom in the atria, appear as small, grayish foci of irregular size. Consequently, the myocardium may have a somewhat striped appearance. In skeletal muscles, lesions similar to those in the myocardium may be observed. Sharply delineated areas of necrosis are seen grossly as gray foci of various sizes and microscopically as necrosis of muscle bundles associated with rather intense leukocytic infiltration.

DIAGNOSIS

The characteristic appearance of vesicles in the mouth and on the feet of animals usually narrows the diagnostic possibilities to two or three viral diseases. In the United States, three viruses must be differentiated in vesicular diseases of swine, and in cattle, two viruses must be considered. The determination of susceptibility in three or four species of animals is the first step in positive diagnosis. Those species used in such a test and their susceptibility to the three viruses are presented in Table 8-1.

Differential filtration in the laboratory may aid in distinguishing foot-and-mouth disease and vesicular stomatitis viruses because elementary bodies of vesicular stomatitis are about 10 times the size of the foot-and-mouth virus. The fact that vesicular stomatitis virus can be cultivated in chicken embryos and foot-and-mouth virus cannot is useful in diagnosis. The virus of foot-and-mouth disease regularly

TABLE 8-1. Species Susceptibility to Vesicular Viruses.

Disease	Cattle	Swine	Horses	Guinea pigs
Foot-and-mouth	+ + +	+ +	−	+ +
Vesicular stomatitis	+ +	+ +	+ + +	+ +
Vesicular exanthema	−	+ + +	±	−

produces typical lesions following intramuscular inoculation into a susceptible calf, whereas the intramuscular inoculation of vesicular stomatitis virus fails to do so. Cross-immunity or complement-fixation tests must be made to determine the strain of the virus causing an outbreak. In addition to vesicular stomatitis and vesicular exanthema, other diseases, such as rinderpest, mucosal disease, bluetongue, cowpox, and contagious ecthyma in sheep, are suggestive of foot-and-mouth disease at times.

CONTROL

Foot-and-mouth disease is endemic in many countries of the world, and the prognosis depends on the severity of the disease. It generally has a benign character, and in most instances, the mortality is not high, seldom averaging more than 3% and often less than 1%. The death rate among young stock is higher than among adults and is somewhat greater in young pigs than in calves. The death rate among sheep and goats is usually low. Prognosis is not of much concern in the United States because all exposed animals are slaughtered.

Formerly, there were only two important methods to control foot-and-mouth disease: (1) isolation, quarantine, and disinfection of premises, and (2) slaughter and burial of infected and exposed animals. Slaughter, however, has seldom been used in countries subjected to epizootics, and many countries depend largely on vaccines to control the disease. A complete eradication method consists of complete isolation of the infected premises, prompt slaughter and proper disposal of infected animals, thorough cleansing

and disinfection of premises and all equipment, immediate quarantine of an area of 5 to 50 miles around the infected premises, and periodic inspections coordinated among federal, state, and local authorities. Treatment alleviates the signs of the disease, but does not prevent the spread of infection and interferes with attempts to eradicate the disease. Treatment, therefore, has no place in an eradication program.

Natural immunity in cattle and swine is negligible, although some individuals have greater resistance than others. The new types of viruses and the variations among types may have resulted through the use of vaccines that imperfectly immunized animals, thus setting up within them the means for forcing variations in the field strains. Animals that recover from foot-and-mouth disease caused by a particular type of the virus generally are sufficiently resistant to that type to withstand additional exposure for 4 months to 1 year. They may, however, be immediately infected with one of the other types and thus exhibit typical symptoms of foot-and-mouth disease.

Susceptible animals may be given a measure of passive immunity to foot-and-mouth disease by injection with immune serum just before, or simultaneously with, exposure to the virus. Such protection is short lived, lasting only 1 to 2 weeks, and often is not sufficient to prevent clinical signs. Animals infected with foot-and-mouth disease may also get a so-called passive immunity in emergency situations by injection of material prepared from lymph, blood, or tissues containing the virus and treated chemically or by heating. The resulting immunity, however, is of a limited character, and the inoculations must be repeated frequently.

Of the vaccines used to control foot-and-mouth disease, the most commonly used was developed in Germany just before World War II. Essentially, it consists of the virus adsorbed on aluminum hydroxide, inactivated by formalin, and incubated. Variations of the vaccine have been used in different parts of the world. Generally, the virus for the vaccine is derived from the tongue epithelium of artificially inoculated cattle. Anybody using the vaccine must know the type of virus prevalent in the outbreak. Vaccines must be critically tested to prove that they do not produce, but do protect against, the disease. There is also some evidence that hogs and sheep are not satisfactorily immunized with vaccine made with virus of bovine origin.

Human beings are only slightly susceptible to the virus of foot-and-mouth disease. There have been no recognized cases of human infections in any of the recent outbreaks of the disease in Mexico and Canada, but in the recent outbreak in England, several cases were diagnosed because countless people had close contact with active strains of the virus. Human beings are usually affected by drinking milk from infected animals, and laboratory workers may be accidentally infected through handling the virus.

The symptoms in man are fever, vomiting, a sense of heat and dryness in the mouth, and the appearance of small vesicles on the lips, tongue, and cheeks. Lesions on the hands have also been described. The course of the disease is short, and there are no records of serious complications or deaths.

In the United States, treatment of foot-and-mouth disease is strictly forbidden. Under federal law, all infected and exposed animals must be slaughtered and the carcasses destroyed. The use of immune sera and vaccines is also expressly forbidden. The only acceptable procedure is complete eradication, even though drastic and costly.

African Horse Sickness

African horse sickness is one of the major infectious diseases with which stockmen in Africa must contend. Outbreaks in the Middle East, Asia, and Europe have made it a disease of worldwide significance.

African horse sickness is an old disease. References to it were made in parts of Africa as early as the second century A.D. Evidence that the virus existed in an unidentified reservoir host became apparent when the first horses to exist in the area of the Cape of Good Hope were afflicted in epidemic proportions. The worst outbreak on record occurred in 1854, when some 70,000 horses out of 160,000 in the Cape of Good Hope reportedly died of the disease.

More recently, severe outbreaks occurred in 1914, 1918, 1923, 1940, 1946, and 1953. In 1959, the disease appeared in Iran, Pakistan, and Afghanistan. It spread to India, Turkey, Cypress, Iraq, Syria, Lebanon, and Jordan in 1960, causing a loss of 300,000 Equidae.

African horse sickness appears capable of existing permanently in any area of the world where the principal insect vector, Culicoides, is found. It has been reported that 36 horses died, 220 were destroyed, and 20,000 were vaccinated in southern Spain in the summer of 1966 because of African horse sickness. That was the first recorded appearance of the disease in Europe. Ten thousand animals have died during subsequent outbreaks in Morocco and 250,000 have been vaccinated. United States quarantine officials and veterinarians are constantly on the alert to prevent the introduction of African horse sickness into this country.

A seasonal, insect-borne viral disease enzootic to Africa, African horse sickness is noted chiefly for the high mortality (up to 90%) it causes in horses. The principal vector is a species of tiny gnats, the Culicoides. The virus is harbored in an unknown reservoir host even in the absence of any of the equine species.

The disease has been known to occur in dogs fed meat from infected horses. There is no other public-health significance; African horse sickness does not affect humans.

CAUSE

The causative agent of African horse sickness is a pantropic double-stranded RNA virus found in the blood, tissue fluids, serous exudates, and various internal organs of equines. It is found in the blood from the onset of the febrile reaction. The virus attaches itself to the cells and cannot be separated from them. Forty-two strains of the virus, round in shape and all about 50 mμ in size, have been identified and placed into nine antigenic groups. The virus is moderately resistant to drying and heating, but retains infectivity for many months when stored in a refrigerator without preservatives.

The natural occurrence of African horse sickness in the enzootic areas of Africa is seasonal, appearing usually in the late summer and disappearing after the first frost. In most instances, the outbreaks are preceded by abnormally high rainfall, which apparently creates highly favorable conditions for the development of the insect vector of the virus reservoir. As a general rule, the relatively lower-lying parts of a given area are most severely infected.

FACTORS INFLUENCING SUSCEPTIBILITY

The equine is the only animal naturally affected by this virus. Mules are considerably less susceptible than horses, and infection is rare in donkeys. Experimentally, horses can be readily infected by small injections of virulent blood, tissue emulsions, or bronchial secretions. African horse sickness is not directly contagious; therefore, affected animals placed in stables with susceptible horses do not cause outbreaks of the disease. All available evidence points to biting flies as the natural vectors, but thus far only the Culicoides gnat has been widely incriminated. In areas of enzootic infection, horses protected from Culicoides do not contract the disease.

All horses are susceptible regardless of age, condition, or previous experience with the disease. Because of the various types of virus, a horse may recover from one type only to become ill with another. Usually, the second attack is milder than the first.

TRANSMISSION

Horses do not retain the virus for more than 30 days after recovery from the clinical manifestations of the disease, and there is no evidence that recovered animals play any part in the carry-over of the infection from season to season. The virus is apparently maintained during the winter in a reservoir host confined to the recognized area of distribution of the disease. Extensive transmission experiments from a variety of wild animals, birds, and amphibians caught at random in areas of enzootic African horse sickness produced negative results. However, the disease was transmitted experimentally to a horse by the bites of Aedes aegypti mosquitoes that had been fed a virus suspension. A nonvaccinated yearling horse, obtained from an insect-proof stable, was exposed to 10 mosquitoes during a 7-hour period. Nine of the mosquitoes bit the horse. Six days later, fever was present and swelling of the eyelids was evident. The horse died 18 days after exposure.

The Culicoides gnat has worldwide distribution, yet the disease occurs principally in Africa. Horses from South Africa introduced into Madagascar did not precipitate an outbreak of the disease, although the Culicoides gnat is present on that island. The fact that African horse sickness has occurred in horses introduced into areas where horses, mules, and donkeys have been excluded for many years also points to the probability that the virus is maintained in some nonequine host. The infection in the horse seems to be purely a matter of choice. Once the first infection occurs, horse-to-horse transmission readily results. Infected animals moved into areas free of African horse sickness easily provide a focus for transmission of the disease through native gnat vectors.

SIGNS

The signs of African horse sickness are variable (Fig. 8-2) because there are four forms of the disease. The incubation period is generally 5 to 7 days, though it may be shorter or longer. An intermittent temperature reaching 104 to 106° F 24 to 72 hours after onset is common in all forms.

Pulmonary or Acute Form

This form is commonly seen in current virulent outbreaks. Distinct signs of respiratory difficulty appear within 3 to 4 days of infection with a temperature rise to 105 to 106° F. The appetite remains good, even after severe coughing develops. As the disease progresses, the animal is seized by fits of coughing and may discharge large quantities of yellowish serous fluid and froth. It stands with head and neck distended and ears drooped, and it sweats severely. Finally, it may choke, then sway, stagger, and fall. The voluminous discharge of fluid indicates that the animal drowns in its own fluids. In rare instances, less severe symptoms occur; the animal

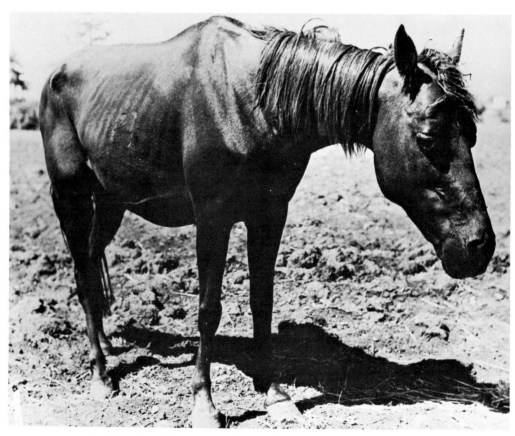

Fig. 8–2.   General appearance of horse suffering from African horse sickness.

recovers but experiences difficulty in breathing for some time after the other signs disappear.

Cardiac Form

The cardiac form is the subacute form of the disease. The incubation period may be as long as 3 weeks. The rise in temperature generally occurs more slowly and persists for a longer period than in the pulmonary form. The most evident signs are distinct swellings of the temporal fossae (area above the eyes) and edema of the eyelids and lips. Hemorrhages may also develop on the eye membranes. In fatal cases, there are distinct signs of heart failure; the heart sac may be partially filled with fluid. The recovery rate from the cardiac form is higher than that from the pulmonary form.

Mixed Form

The clinical signs of this form are a combination of the signs of the cardiac and pulmonary forms. Although the signs of either may be more prominent, both pulmonary and cardiac lesions are found by necropsy. The incubation period is usually between 5 and 7 days. An infected horse will probably recover if it is still alive 5 days after the onset of clinical signs.

Horse Sickness Fever

This form of the disease is mild, and the incubation period varies from 5 days to a month. Signs are slight. The only indications of infection may be a brief rise in temperature to 105° F, slight conjunctivitis, an accelerated pulse, some loss of appetite, and slightly labored breathing. This form is generally seen in horses undergoing immunization, and recovery is usually rapid.

DIAGNOSIS

In the severe forms of the disease, the course is rarely longer than 5 days because the animal dies within that time. In milder forms, the course may be several weeks.

With outbreaks of African horse sickness in the Middle East, Europe, and parts of Asia, locale can no longer be relied on as a factor in diagnosis. In enzootic areas, familiarity with the gross signs and lesions makes quick diagnosis possible. However, because of the many viral strains and the various forms of the disease, a confirming laboratory diagnosis is essential. This is usually done by serum neutralization tests and is similar in principle to the toxin-antitoxin reaction.

TREATMENT AND CONTROL

As might be expected, no form of specific therapy has been successful in the treatment of African horse sickness. Upon recognition of the disease, infected animals should be slaughtered and buried.

Prophylactic immunization has been accepted as an indispensable aid to the control of African horse sickness. A polyvalent vaccine made from the nine separate viral serotypes found in Africa and the Middle East provides protection for as long as 5 years. The immunity is not permanent, and exposed animals should be vaccinated annually before the horse sickness season.

Vaccine is produced by intracerebral passage through mice. With serial passage in this species, neurotropic adaptation of the virus occurs. (Virus adapts itself to nervous tissue.) By the hundredth passage, the virus becomes attenuated to the point where it may be injected into horses with almost complete safety. Immune mares convey a passive immunity to their foals, protecting them until after weaning.

In addition to vaccination, susceptible animals should be protected from nocturnal biting insects by stabling and insecticides and by grazing on high-lying pastures away from rivers, streams, or wet ground. Good control practice involves treating ponds, lakes, slow-moving water, and other breeding places of gnats in an affected area.

Movement of animals from known areas of infection should be restricted. The extensive spread of the disease in the Middle East and Asia since 1959 provides evidence of the problems involved in confinement. There is little possibility of intercontinental introduction of the disease through shipments of horses vaccinated and quarantined in insect-proof stables before and after shipment. However, because of the speed of modern means of transportation, the infected vector may be transmitted by airplane; this is probably the way the infection reached the Middle East.

Because the present experience in Asia and Europe indicates that the disease cannot readily be eradicated even by intensive application of effective vaccination, the solution to control lies in the identification of the unknown virus reservoir. Although this may not simplify control of the disease in enzootic areas, it may be extremely valuable in preventing its spread into countries that at present, are free of African horse sickness.

CHAPTER 9
Diseases Caused by Poisonous Substances

Two potential harmful effects can occur when a food animal ingests, inhales, or is otherwise exposed to a poisonous substance. The first is the effect on the life of the animal and the second is the effect on the consumer of the residue of the substance in the animal if the animal or its products enter the food chain.

RECOMMENDED READING

Amstutz, HE: Bovine Medicine and Surgery. 2nd Edition. Chap. 8. Santa Barbara, CA, American Veterinary Publications, 1980.

Buck, WB, and Osweiler, GD: Clinical and Diagnostic Veterinary Toxicology. 2nd Edition. Dubuque, IA, Kendall/Hunt, 1976.

Kingsberry, JM: Poisonous Plants of the U.S. and Canada. Englewood Cliffs, Prentice-Hall, 1964.

Clark, EGC, and Clark, ML: Veterinary Toxicology. Philadelphia, Lea & Febiger, 1975.

Poisonous Plants

Toxicological problems are difficult to prevent because there are many poisonous substances to consider. The poison may be a naturally occurring plant constituent or a chemical introduced into and not normally found in the natural environment. When diagnosing poisonings it is helpful to examine the entire herd, observing the animals for any deviation from normal, while evaluating all known facts surrounding the problem. Pastures should be examined for poisonous plants, discarded paint buckets, fertilizer spills, and other possible sources of poisoning. Overgrazing of pastures and ranges is probably the greatest single factor in losses from poisonous plants.

Livestock producers must consider their management procedures and shortcomings when multiple poisonings occur on a property because most incidences are the result of carelessness, poor management, or ignorance.

On most properties, the prevention of plant poisoning is, in general, a matter of livestock and pasture management. The main step is the eradication of poisonous plants from all parts of the property. If the farm is in a prairie region, such eradication is relatively easy. If the farm includes woodland, natural meadows, or other areas where native plant life persists, the problem is more difficult. The farmer must, then, know poisonous plants, keep the number of them as small as possible, and keep animals away from them during seasons when they may be eaten in quantity. Most poisonous plants are weeds and can be eradicated by the general practices used for weeds. When complete eradication is impossible, more must be known about poisonous plants—the stages at which they are poisonous, the seasons when they are dangerous, and the conditions under which they cause poisoning. Valuable animals can then be prevented from feeding on them.

Poisonous plants are a hazard to livestock in many native pastures when the right set of circumstances occurs. Generally, most plant poisonings occur early in the spring before grass is adequate, or during periods of drought when green feed is scarce. The toxic substance of some plants is concentrated in the young growing leaves in the spring, whereas in other plants, the toxic substance is found in the seeds and stems later in the season.

Generally, only a few poisonous plants are troublesome in an area, and producers should learn to recognize them. Bulletins or books are available from the state agricultural extension services.

HYDROCYANIC ACID POISONING

This poisoning can occur from several plants, such as arrow grass, Johnson grass, Sudan grass, common sorghum, wild black cherry, chokeberry, pin cherry, and flax. All these plants contain cyanogenetic glycosides, which, when hydrolyzed by enzymes in the digestive tract, yield hydrocyanic acid (prussic acid).

Johnson grass and Sudan grass are considered good pasture grasses, but when normal growth is interrupted by drought, frost, trampling, or other causes, hydrocyanic acid may develop to a point where the plants become toxic to livestock. The cyanogenetic glycoside content is increased by heavy nitrate fertilization and excessive irrigation or heavy rainfall. Very young, rapidly growing plants are most hazardous. Neither freezing nor wilting increases the glycoside content, but both tend to increase the free hydrocyanic acid content, resulting in a temporary increase in toxicity.

Sheep and cattle may be poisoned by eating arrow grass, the leaves of which contain hydrocyanic or prussic acid. Species of arrow grass that poison livestock are widely distributed in marshy pastures and native grass-hay areas throughout the United States. When arrow grass has adequate moisture, it does not cause poisoning; when growth is stunted from lack of moisture or an early frost, however, plants quickly become toxic. Arrow grass grows best in soil covered with water and, in such soil, may spread over large areas. It sometimes grows in small patches in moist soil or near springs.

About $1/50$ of an ounce of hydrocyanic acid (¼ to 3 pounds of stunted arrow grass) will kill a 600-pound animal. The toxic dose must be eaten at one time to cause death because the poison is not cumulative. Death results from respiratory failure.

Signs of poisoning are: nervousness, abnormal breathing (either rapid or slow and deep), trembling or jerking muscles, reddened coloration of the lining of the mouth, and spasms or convulsions continuing at short intervals until respiratory failure causes death.

BRACKEN FERN POISONING

This fern is widely distributed in North America. When ingested by cattle and sheep it causes cumulative poisoning, which takes from 1 to 3 weeks to develop. Signs of poisoning may occur for 2 weeks or more after animals have been removed from fern foliage. Cases generally develop in late summer or fall following periods of drought.

Sheep and cattle show toxic signs after eating green ferns daily for a period of time. Cattle have hemorrhages in various parts of their bodies, develop a fever, and lose weight rapidly. They are affected by the so-called aplastic anemia factor, which depresses bone marrow function. The poisoning is irreversible. The onset of signs is sudden and of short duration, and death loss may approach 90% of those affected. Treatment should be initiated under the direction of the local veterinarian, although few cattle recover after signs of acute poisoning appear.

Animals seldom eat bracken fern if sufficient forage is available. To eliminate livestock losses, do not overgraze ranges. Be sure sufficient forage is available at all times to animals in infested areas. If necessary, give supplement near the end of the grazing period. Without supplement, animals often eat toxic amounts of bracken to make up for the decreased nutrient value of mature plants.

Bracken fern can be eradicated. In areas where cultivation is practical, the plants can be destroyed by cultivating the soil for 2 to 3 years. Keeping the tops cut starves the roots and prevents spread.

CROOKED-CALF DISEASE

Toxic species of lupine weed eaten by cows during early pregnancy cause crooked-calf disease, a crippling disorder of calves that is present at birth.

Stricken calves have twisted and badly aligned leg bones, twisted backs or necks, or cleft palates. One or more of these defects can cause handicaps ranging from an inability to move or eat to harmless bone alterations noticeable only on x-ray films.

Lupine, or beanweed, is a plant of the pea family with multiple leaflets radiating in a finger-like manner from a common point. A spike of white, pink, yellow, or bluish florets projects from the top. Only a few of the more than 100 known species have thus far been found toxic. Lupine grows on foothills and mountain ranges in many areas of the west. The poisonous species are perennials, although some lupines are annuals. Poisonous species are dangerous from the time they start to grow in the spring until they dry up in the fall; most are especially dangerous during the seed stage in late summer. Pods and seeds retain their toxicity even when the plants are matured.

Cows that graze on toxic lupines may show moderate reactions. They exhibit a reluctance to move and a stiff-legged walk; coats are rough, noses are dry, and feces are hard. In many instances, these cows later produce deformed calves. There is no direct relation between severity of symptoms in the mother and severity of deformity in the offspring. Cattle are often poisoned by eating 1 to 2 pounds of lupine without other forage.

Comparison of cows fed lupine during various stages of early pregnancy showed that the worst time for grazing on contaminated ranges was between the fortieth and seventieth days of pregnancy. Slight to moderate bone malformation, however, resulted during experimental feed trials when cows ate lupine after that time span.

Unfortunately, cows are likely to eat lupine at the critical time (August) when most of the herd is 1 or 2 months' pregnant, range pastures tend to dry up, and good feed becomes scarce. Cattle normally do not like lupine, but they eat it when there is no other choice. The best way for ranchers to avoid crooked-calf disease is to provide an alternative to lupine ranges, at least during the first 120 days of pregnancy.

Losses may be heavy when hungry sheep are trailed through lupine ranges in the late summer. Supplemental feeding is helpful at such times.

SWEET-CLOVER POISONING

Sweet clover, a valuable forage crop, may be used freely as pasture, but the feeding of damaged or spoiled sweet-clover hay or silage may cause death. Death losses from sweet-clover poisoning in a herd may vary from 1 or 2 animals to 15 or 20 animals.

Prior to the isolation of dicumarol, the hemorrhagic agent in spoiled sweet-clover hay, an infectious agent was considered as a possible cause of the condition. The appearance of the signs suggests a transmissible infectious disease because the condition occurs simultaneously in several animals on the same farm. Additionally, in feeding trials, the disease appeared in cattle of the same age and after approximately the same length of time.

Dicumarol has been isolated from experimentally produced spoiled hays and from hays fatal to cattle in field cases. The substance is insoluble in acid media but forms salts in basic or alkaline solutions. The damaged hay is usually moldy, but not all moldy hay is poisonous. Dicumarol poisoning is usually seen in winter after cattle have been fed damaged sweet-clover hay for approximately 2 weeks.

In sweet-clover poisoning, nothing in the appearance of cattle attracts attention until hemorrhages occur. Swellings representing subcutaneous hemorrhage are usually noticed first. The swelling is often great enough to cause lameness.

The mucosa are pale, and persistent bleeding occurs from superficial cuts and scratches. Progressive weakness follows anemia resulting from loss of blood. Affected cattle may remain bright and alert and may continue to ruminate. Unless pressure from hemorrhage blocks the esophagus and stops eructation, bloating does not occur. With the hemorrhaging, the heart rate quickens, and the increased force of the beat is obvious. Death results from anemia.

Animals dehorned or castrated while in the toxic state bleed to death because coagulation is inhibited. Bleeding is particularly severe during parturition if toxicity is present; both the dam and calf usually die.

Calves are more susceptible to the disease than are older cattle, but mature animals may show signs of the condition if the spoiled hay is fed to them over a sufficiently long period. Because of their physiologic deficiency of vitamin K, newborn animals and infants are particularly sensitive to the anticoagulant. Lactating animals, however, are usually resistant to the toxic substance. The drug passes the placental barrier; this is shown by the fact that the prothrombin level is reduced in newborn animals from dams fed spoiled sweet-clover hay.

The characteristic lesion is hemorrhage into the tissue in all parts of the body. Blood in the tissues usually clots after death occurs, but blood in the peritoneal cavity remains fluid. The hemorrhages are found most often in the subcutaneous tissues and intermuscular fascia, but lesions have been seen in the brain and in the medullary cavities of the long bones.

There is much variation in the time required to produce sweet-clover toxicity, thus indicating that all damaged clover hay is not equally toxic. Coagulation of the blood is not usually retarded before 14 days of feeding moldy hay; the average time is about 15 days. If coagulation has not been adversely affected within 3 weeks, the hay is probably not highly toxic and the onset of hemorrhaging will not occur until after about 30 days. Toxic hay does not lose its toxicity, and experiments have shown that it can cause hemorrhage after 4 years in storage.

Herd history may immediately suggest a diagnosis of sweet-clover poisoning, or careful examination of affected animals and necropsies may be necessary to confirm the diagnosis. Sweet-clover disease should be suspected when sudden deaths occur in cattle fed on sweet-clover hay or when several animals die within a day or two after dehorning or castrating. Upon postmortem examination, excessive hemorrhages should substantiate the diagnosis of sweet-clover disease.

Properly cured sweet clover is not toxic and is a good feed, although it is unpalatable because of the woody fiber of its stems. Sweet clover is not toxic when grazed and can be used economically in this manner.

Cattle alternately fed good hay and toxic sweet-clover hay may not be affected, depending on the toxicity of the hay and the ratio of substitution. With highly toxic hay, a 50:50 ratio may still produce the disease. If sweet clover is fed until a delay in clotting time becomes apparent, and a safe forage is then fed, trouble is not likely to be encountered.

FESCUE FOOT

Cattle feeding on tall fescue, a valuable pasture grass, occasionally develop lameness. The disease in cattle is peculiar in that the signs of lameness first appear in the left hind foot in a great number of animals. Fescue foot is thought to be caused by either toxins produced by the plant or a fungus. The exact cause is not known.

All breeds of cattle are susceptible to the condition, which resembles chronic ergotism but has a predilection for the feet. The poisoning may appear as an outbreak, and many cattle on improperly managed pastures may be affected during droughts. When the grass has received little fertilizer or has not been previously grazed or mowed, it is of poor quality in late fall and winter. Cattle grazing on it are subject to extreme malnutrition if supplemental feed is not provided. Fescue foot is prevalent in animals suffering from malnutrition and also occurs in cattle fed fescue hay or silage.

On the other hand, few cases of fescue foot have been reported in cattle rotated on well-managed pastures of fescue-legume mixture or of vigorously growing stands of pure fescue.

The disease may appear 10 days to several weeks after cattle start to feed on fescue; they are most susceptible to fescue foot when first placed on fescue pasture.

Usually, the first clinical signs are general stiffness and soreness. Affected cattle are slow to move and refuse to graze. They become dull and listless as their rate of breathing increases. They lose weight rapidly. Cattle soon become lame in the hind feet. Hooves may split.

At this time, fescue foot may be confused with foot rot. Cattle with foot rot usually develop distinct swelling and inflammation in the space between the claws. There is no such swelling in fescue foot.

As fescue foot progresses, dry gangrene develops in the foot tissues. Skin around the hoof breaks; a definite line marks the affected area. In severe cases, sloughing of foot tissue occurs at this time. Also, the switch, the end of the tail, and, in rare instances, the tip of the ears may slough off.

No medication is effective for cattle with fescue foot. In severe cases where sloughing has occurred, animals should be destroyed for humane reasons.

Cattle usually recover completely if they are removed from fescue pasture or fescue hay and are given other feed as soon as the first signs of the disease appear. After they recover, cattle may be safely returned to fescue pasture if the grass is growing satisfactorily. These cattle should be checked daily for signs of recurrence.

Proper management of fescue pasture is the best way to prevent fescue foot. Pasture rotation helps to prevent fescue foot during severe drought when forage is badly needed. The following procedure is recommended for rotating pastures.

1. Put cattle on other forage for 10 days.
2. Follow with fescue pasture for the next 10 days.
3. Continue pasture rotation at 10-day intervals until the drought breaks.

Tall fescue is adapted to many soils and climates in the United States. Because it grows well on soils of low productivity, this pasture grass has made a major contribution to the agriculture of the south central and southeastern states. The grass may be maintained in legume-fescue mixtures or in pure stands. When fescue pasture is fertilized and well managed, cattle make satisfactory gains. On pure stands of fescue, young cattle gain 0.8 to 1.5 pounds a day. Cattle on legume-fescue mixtures make gains comparable to gains achieved on other cool-season legume-grass mixtures.

Cattle that are grazing fescue should be provided for free choice with adequate amounts of salt, bone meal, limestone and, perhaps, a mineral supplement containing minor elements.

GRASS-SEED NEMATODE POISONING

Grass-seed nematode poisoning of animals is a sporadic condition difficult to diagnose because the principal clinical sign is nervousness, followed shortly by death. The condition occurs where grasses are subject to the grass-seed nematode disease caused by the larval stages of Anguina agrostis. The grass seeds in only two diseases, ergot and grass-seed nematode disease, are replaced by sclerotia and galls toxic to livestock. The effects of ergot poisoning on livestock are well documented, but little is known about grass-seed nematode poisoning.

The clinical signs in cattle are neuromuscular, such as knuckling of the forefeet, lowering of the head between the forelegs, sweating, staggering, falling, convulsions, and death. In dairy cattle, the first sign is a drop in milk production, followed by the other symptoms if the toxic hay is not removed.

Farmers in central Oregon produce a variety of seed crops, and they customarily feed the seed screenings to livestock in the winter months. The seed screenings resulting from the cleaning of Chewings fescue seed contain a large proportion of seed galls. The seed galls contain many larval nematodes, which leave the galls after wet weather in the spring and migrate to the grass leaves. When the grass panicles develop, the microscopic nematodes penetrate the ovaries and stimulate the plant to produce galls. In any seed head, one or all of the seeds may be affected.

The infested seeds contain a heat-stable, alcohol-soluble substance that is toxic to livestock when added to their normal diet.

Many grasses may be infested sporadically by A. agrostis. Among these grasses are Chewings fescue, creeping red fescue, Kentucky bluegrass, annual bluegrass, velvet grass, sweet vernal grass, creeping timothy, red top, spike bent, highland bent grass, velvet bent grass, seaside bent grass, orchard grass, and buffalo grass.

Wheat and rye are infested by another species of this genus, Anguina tritici, but it is not known if this nematode is toxic to animals. In wheat, the nematode causes the formation of gall in place of the grain. The galls are shorter than the wheat grains and look like smut balls. However, the galls are hard, whereas the smut balls are soft and easily crushed with the fingers. In addition, other related nematode species infest seeds sporadically in species of Calamagrostis, Danthonia, Elymus, Holcus, Sporobolus, and Stipa throughout the country.

The disease in grass plants may be controlled only by drastic measures and by constant attention to prevent a recurrence. Effective measures include burning of fescue fields following the harvest of seeds to destroy galls in the stubble, rotation of crops for several years, and use of costly chemicals. (The grass-seed nematode disease involves only the seed heads so that the grass may be utilized for lawn or turf.)

Poisonous Minerals and Mixtures

UREA POISONING

More than half of all cattle in feedlots in the United States are probably fed some urea, according to findings of a survey reported by the United States Department of Agriculture covering more than 6000 cattle feeders.

Urea is fed in commercial mixed feed, in a concentrate ration mixed by the cattle feeder or to his order, or in silage.

Until recently, the urea used in livestock feed was difficult to measure. Urea is widely used for fertilizer and industrial purposes as well as for feed, and technical problems formerly restricted feed use to "feed-grade" urea. However, these problems have largely been solved, and most commercial grades of urea have become multipurpose in use. Thus, commonly quoted estimates of feed-grade urea represent only part of the urea actually fed to livestock.

More than half of all feedlot operators who buy urea as a separate ingredient mix it on the farm with their own equipment. Local feed dealers mix for small feedlots.

Some guidelines for feeding urea to beef cattle are:

1. Do not feed urea or supplements containing urea to newly arrived or shipped-in cattle for a period of 21 to 28 days, or to cattle that have been starved or off feed for 36 hours until they have had a chance to fill up with feed.

2. Feed a maximum of 0.15 pound of urea daily to growing or wintering cattle.

3. Feed no more than 0.22 pound of urea per head daily to fattening steers or heifers on grain and roughage.

4. Do not feed urea to young calves until after the rumen develops—at about 6 to 8 weeks of age.

5. Formulate complete cattle rations so that no more than 33% of the crude protein or nitrogen is derived from urea.

6. Do not feed urea over and above the protein requirements.

7. Mix urea in a properly balanced supplement or a complete ration; do not feed free-choice or self-feed urea supplements.

The recommendations for use of urea in dairy cattle are not as clearcut as those for beef cattle because there is a variation in the level of grain fed for different levels of milk production. Urea can be used to replace as much as 35% of the protein of the concentrate ration of dairy cattle after rumen function has been established. A high-urea protein supplement, as much as 20% of urea or 90% of the protein from urea, can be used, but it should be mixed in the ration so that the urea level does not exceed recommended allowances.

Urea is used by rumen microorganisms and supplies nitrogen for the synthesis of amino acids. Amino acids are eventually either incorporated into tissue protein or used to form ammonia. In the first process, the animal makes its own protein from a relatively inexpensive material. In the second, the nitrogen is not only largely wasted, but the product is toxic and absorbed into the blood.

The toxicity of urea largely depends on the energy content of the ration, the kinds of microorganisms making up the rumen flora, and the rate of consumption of urea. The rumen may be conditioned to convert urea to amino acids rather than to ammonia by starting at a low level and gradually increasing the amount fed. This presumably encourages multiplication of bacteria that synthesize amino acids at the expense of those that do not. One hundred grams of urea in a single feeding will kill a 1000-pound cow not previously fed urea. The same amount distributed over two or three feedings will not be lethal because the ammonia concentration in the blood will remain below a critical level.

Under feedlot conditions, as much as 300 g of urea per day per 1000-lb animal may be fed to cows adapted to urea feeding. (Note, however, that renal damage may result at this high level.) When animals are kept off feed for a short time, even 24 to 48 hours, they lose much of their adaptability to urea and may be killed by the same level they had earlier consumed safely.

The clinical signs of urea toxicity in cattle are severe groaning, shivering, staggering, labored rapid breathing, violent struggling, and death.

NITRATE-NITRITE POISONING

Nitrate poisoning is often the consequence of a complex of mismanagement. It can result from careless handling of fertilizers or other nitrate-containing chemical mixtures or from the accidental ingestion of the chemicals. Secondly, animals may graze on pastures or ranges where nitrate-bearing plants are prevalent. Thirdly, the poisoning may result from drinking water, either from naturally nitrate-bearing springs or from streams, ponds, or wells contaminated with nitrate-bearing run-off water.

Perhaps this problem is becoming more important because of recent innovations and trends in modern agriculture. Natural waterways and surface drainage undoubtedly contain more nitrates leeched from surface applications of fertilizer products. Surface contamination from feedlot drainage, old manure piles, and other sources is an important factor, especially in poorly placed farm wells.

Geologic surveys and public-health surveys have shown that natural spring waters and wells less than 200 feet deep often contain levels of nitrate hazardous to animal and human health. Reports show that some wells in Minnesota have a nitrate-nitrogen content of 190 ppm. Under some circumstances, this content approaches the minimum lethal amount for swine. Some wells in Missouri and Kansas show a content of more than 800 ppm. Such sources of water should not be used for any human or animal consumption.

Most water analyses are based on nitrate level. One must remember that swine can tolerate large amounts of nitrate, but are highly susceptible to nitrite. This susceptibility introduces an additional hazard to the swine industry, because nitrate can be converted to nitrite by bacterial action, especially by organisms of the coliform group that abound at or near livestock sources of water. Zinc from storage tanks, coated water lines, and waterers also act as conversion agents.

During the growing season, plants absorb nitrate from the soil; the nitrate is reduced in nitrite in the stems and leaves. Continuous nitrate absorption from the soil, coupled with retarded growth, may lead to nitrate or nitrite concentration because of incomplete reduction. (Examples of conditions leading to retarded growth include drought, shade, herbicide action, and plant disease or injury.) Accelerated nitrate absorption following rainfall—especially after a period of drought—may also cause such concentration, and heavy nitrate fertilization adds to the problem. Under such conditions, immature plants in particular tend to concentrate nitrate or nitrite.

Nitrate concentrations in silage are reduced, but not eliminated, by the fermentation process. Silage forages containing moderate amounts of nitrate can be fed safely if offered in small amounts over a long period of time. In ruminant animals, carbohydrates hasten the conversion of nitrate into amino acids, hence reducing the toxic effects of excess nitrate in the feed. Feeding roughage containing nitrates should be supplemented with vitamin A. Remember that small amounts of nitrate may affect feed utilization without causing clinical signs of toxicity.

In cattle, symptoms of nitrate toxicity are a marked drop in milk flow within a week after chopped hay or silage is fed, increased urine production that is darker than normal, and apparent digestive failures. In a type of toxicity that appears slowly, milk flow declines and symptoms of vitamin A deficiency appear. When abortions are noted, they usually occur in the third to fifth month.

Abnormal births are common, and calves carried to term are born dead or die immediately after birth. Nitrate-bearing oat hay and corn-stalk poisoning appear to act similarly, in that sudden losses may occur when cattle or sheep ingest nitrates.

Chemically, the nitrates are converted to nitrites in the rumen. The resulting nitrites compete with the oxygen, tying up the erythrocyte-oxygen mechanism in the blood. Blood from these animals is chocolate brown. Feedstuffs incriminated in nitrate poisoning are corn silage or fodder; sorghum silage; oat hay or silage; Sudan pasture, hay or silage; and alfalfa hay.

FLUOROSIS

Fluorine is an active chemical element widely distributed in soil, water, rocks, and plants in many parts of the world, but most often encountered in water from deep wells in the more arid parts of this country. Fluorine combines with other elements to form fluorides. Toxic quantities of fluorides occur in a few products used in feeding animals, such as raw rock phosphates and phosphatic limestone.

Chronic fluorosis results from the ingestion of small amounts of fluoride over a long period of time. This occurs primarily where livestock consume water that is high in fluorine and forage that is contaminated with wastes from nearby industrial plants. All types of livestock may be affected by excessive amounts of fluorides, although cattle are the most susceptible (followed by sheep and swine). The severity of the lesions caused by fluorine poisoning depends on the form of the fluoride ingested, the age and species of animal, the nutrient level, the level and period of consumption, and the state of reproduction and lactation.

The clinical signs associated with fluorosis include staining and mottling of the teeth with excessive wearing of the incisors. In severe cases, exostoses may appear at the joints, the shafts of the long bones may thicken, and the animal may exhibit intermittent lameness. Acute fluoride poisoning is characterized by diarrhea, sudden loss of appetite, loss of weight, and inflammation of the stomach and intestine.

Prevention of fluorosis depends on recognizing potential sources of consumption of the chemical and eliminating the possibility of excessive intake.

WOOD-PRESERVATIVE POISONING

Pentachlorophenol (penta), a wood preservative, is toxic for swine. Penta itself does not stain wood, but a stain, such as coal tar or creosote, is almost always added. These compounds may be more dangerous than the penta. Arsenic or lead in boiled linseed oil, as an additive, may also constitute a hazard.

Pentachlorophenol is readily absorbed through intact skin and causes increased metabolism, nervousness, rapid respiration, muscle tremors, and death. On contact, it burns the skin and mucous membranes of pigs and irritates the skin of adult swine. Prolonged contact may slow growth in feeder pigs.

Typically afflicted newborn pigs nurse well but become ill with fever, muscle tremors, and labored breathing. Death occurs several hours later. Internal necropsy lesions are usually absent, but the skin may be red where it has come in contact with treated lumber. Survivors develop ulcers of the oral mucosa, knees, and soles of the feet. Reduced food intake and bacterial arthritis may follow.

Though adult swine are more resistant to the effects of penta, some sows become restless and, if not removed from the pen, may become hysterical. Prolonged contact of pregnant sows with penta reportedly causes weak or stillborn pigs. It has also been reported that, if sows are confined to treated farrowing crates for 7 to 10 days before farrowing, newborn pigs may bleed to death via the navel.

In one instance, a boardwalk treated with wood preservative 20 years previously but still in good condition was salvaged to build a slatted floor. Weaned pigs placed on this floor developed blood dyscrasias, and 10% died of hepatitis and anemia. The problem occurred in each group of pigs placed on the floor. Arsenicals and coal tar may have been the poisons in this wood. In another instance, adding sufficient bedding to keep the pigs off the floor, washing with lye soap, and allowing the wood to weather for a year still did not resolve the problem adequately.

LEAD POISONING

Lead poisoning is common in pastured animals. Old paint buckets dumped on trash piles and old batteries on which curious cattle may chew and lick are common causes. Signboards are another source because cattle may make them a loafing place, especially when the rest of the pasture is relatively free of shade.

Buildings that have not been painted for years and appear to be free of paint are often the source of lead poisoning—again because they are loafing areas. The licking of buildings by cattle is likely to occur in winter and early spring months before grass starts or in periods of drought when grass is in short supply.

The lead content on forage and other plants may reach levels toxic to livestock at the edges of heavily traveled highways, especially if some of the common orchard sprays are used to control weeds.

Lead is a cumulative poison, and the toxic effects may not become evident until many small doses have equaled a toxic dose.

The clinical signs of acute lead poisoning appear in animals as two separate, although related, syndromes. The first syndrome is a stage of inflammation caused by the corrosive effect of the metal on the mucous membranes of the stomach and intestines. This leads to loss of appetite, salivation, intestinal pain, grinding of the teeth, and either constipation or diarrhea. The second syndrome involves the effects of the lead on the nervous system. Animals appear deranged, walk in circles, stand with heads pressed against a wall or a tree, and bellow as if frenzied.

In the chronic stage, animals are depressed, lose weight, and stagger when forced to move.

As with most other preventable diseases, the primary means of prevention is good management.

ARSENIC POISONING

Arsenic poisoning probably occurs less frequently now than in years past, but still must be mentioned. Sodium arsenite, lead, and calcium arsenate have been used as herbicides and insecticides, and the improper disposal of dust or spray containers had been a common cause of arsenic poisoning. Newer and safer pesticides have reduced this problem to a great extent.

Arsenic is poisonous to animals both by absorption through the skin and by oral ingestion.

Clinical signs of arsenic poisoning include general weakness, muscle twitching, weak pulse, and staggering gait. Diarrhea is an inevitable sign and results from the destruction of the mucosal lining of the gastrointestinal tract. Because of abdominal pain, animals get up and lie down, kick at the belly, and bite at the flanks. Feces may be copious, watery, and flecked with blood.

Insecticide Poisoning

ORGANIC PHOSPHATE POISONING

The organophosphate compounds are sometimes referred to as the "nerve-gas insecticides" because of the origin of the compounds.

All breeds of livestock are susceptible to poisoning with organophosphate compounds. Neither age nor sex has any significant bearing on susceptibility, but young animals are more sensitive than adults.

Organophosphates may enter the body by inhalation of the vapor, by absorption of the liquid through the skin and eyes, and by ingestion with forage crops or other feedstuffs. However, poisoning usually results from the accidental consumption of an overdose of the insecticide. Inaccurate computation of the oral or dermal dose may cause poisoning. The products are dangerous if improperly used, not only because small doses may be lethal but because sublethal doses are cumulative. All animals exposed to excessive doses should be moved to noncontaminated areas, even when they do not exhibit symptoms.

The clinical signs may be local or systemic in origin and may appear a few minutes or several hours after exposure. The time lag depends to some degree on the specific product, the amount absorbed, and the route of exposure.

Ocular and respiratory effects are caused by conjunctival exposure or inhalation of the insecticide and are evidenced by nasal discharge, prolonged wheezing, rapid respiration, constricted pupils, and, occasionally, protruding tongue.

Systemic signs resulting from absorption of higher concentrations are evidenced by sweating, loss of appetite, respiratory difficulties, muscle twitching, restlessness, depression, convulsions, paralysis, and death.

To avoid poisoning, great care should be exercised when using insecticides or any other external medicament. Read the labels carefully and follow directions explicitly. Most insecticides are toxic, although none is likely to cause poisoning when used strictly according to label directions.

OTHER INSECTICIDE POISONINGS

The signs of poisoning from dichlorodiphenyl trichloroethane (DDT) and methoxychlor are distinctive and easily recognized. The same can be said for other groups or related insecticides; therefore, they are considered in outline form in Table 9-1.

TABLE 9-1. Signs of Chemical Poisoning.

General Signs	Individual Signs	Chemical
Muscular tremors very fine at first, progressing to coarse tremors, to steady shivering. Initiated by stimulant first but constant at later period. Loss of coordination, dyspnea, apprehension, and hypersensitivity.	Hyperirritability Hyperirritability Hyperirritability Hyperirritability Hyperirritability	DDT TDE Methoxychlor Perthane Dilan
Muscular spasms, twitches, jerks or convulsions, no steady tremors but may respond to sudden stimuli. Excessive salivation (mostly frothy). May be depressed but mainly apprehensive and hypersensitive. Onset may be abrupt but recovery sudden.	Odor of rosin or pine. Musty or metallic odor. Aromatic or pleasant odor. Odor absent or not well defined. Odor absent or not well defined. Odor absent or not well defined. Odor absent or not well defined. Odor absent or not well defined. Odor absent or not well defined.	Toxaphene Benzene hexachloride (BHC) or Lindane Chlordane Heptachlor Dieldrin Aldrin Endrin Thiodan Telodrin
Excessive salivation, fluid or stringy, dyspnea, muscular stiffness or weakness, with or without tremors or trembling. Hypersensitivity and apprehension. Often demonstrate extreme nervous signs.	Excessive salivation. Excessive salivation. Excessive salivation. Excessive salivation. Trembling or rage. Abrupt onset, swift recovery. Mild nervous signs. Violent nervous signs. Progressive nervous signs.	Trichlorofon (Dipterex, Neguvon) Dimethyldichlorvinyl phosphate (DDVP, Vapona) Diazinon Tetraethylpyrophosphate (TEPP) Sevin Pyrolan Compound 4072 Ruelene Co-Ral
Great muscular weakness, inapparent until handled, dragging feet, limp tail. May develop dyspnea and excessive salivation.	Diarrhea	Ronnel

CHAPTER 10
Diseases Caused by Parasites

The organism, Anaplasma sp., is included in this chapter because of the type of vector usually involved in transmission of disease. Classified as Rickettsia, some may consider the organism as a parasite of red blood cells. The succeeding sections discussing ecto- and endoparasites are summaries and examples that describe potential control of types of life cycles.

RECOMMENDED READING

Amstutz, HE: Bovine Medicine and Surgery. 2nd Edition. Chap. 5. Santa Barbara, CA, American Veterinary Publications, 1980.

Ivens, VR, Mark, DL, and Levine, NO: Principal Parasites of Domestic Animals in the United States. Special Pub. 52. Urbana-Champaign, Il, University of Illinois at Urbana-Champaign, 1978.

Soulsby, EJL: Helminths, Arthropods and Protozoa of Domesticated Animals. 7th Edition. Philadelphia, Lea & Febiger, 1981.

Anaplasmosis

Anaplasmosis is an infectious and transmissible disease of cattle that has been of prime concern to the beef and dairy industries over the past 50 years. In bovine species, erythrocytes are invaded and destroyed by the causative agents, Anaplasma marginale and Anaplasma centrale, which are protozoa-like microorganisms. This invasion is evidenced biologically by rapidly progressive anemia and jaundice in adult animals and anemia of lesser extent in calves. In recognition of this anemic condition, a more specific designation of *bovine infectious anemia* has been recorded in some veterinary literature.

Historically, the major breakthrough in identifying anaplasmosis as a separate entity occurred in 1883 when workers (Smith and Kilborne) dealing primarily with babesiosis (Texas fever) discovered a new inclusion of the peripheral cytoplasm of erythrocytes. Their findings were published in Bulletin No. 1, Bureau of Animal Industries, United States Department of Agriculture. Further research led to the realization that anaplasmosis was caused by a pathogenic protozoa-like factor and that its invasion of erythrocytes displayed clinical symptoms similar to those of babesiosis. Although anaplasmosis is recognized primarily in semitropical areas, the widespread shipment of cattle, and especially commercial breeding stock, from herds of the southeastern United States has led to the increased incidence of anaplasmosis in more temperate areas of this country.

Endemic areas within the United States have been designated, and correlations with semitropical climatic locations have been found. Heavy morbidity and mortality losses occur in the Gulf coast states and along the Pacific coast, mainly in California. In addition, northern ranges of the Rocky Mountains are recognized as enzootic areas. Prevalence of anaplasmosis in these locales is primarily due to the large arthropod vector population, especially ticks and mites.

CAUSE

The causative agent is a microorganism classified as A. marginale. This nomenclature is justified by the fact that microscopic study demonstrates that the organism is devoid of cytoplasm (literal translation of the term Anaplasma means without cytoplasm). Analyses of infected animals invariably reveal the Anaplasma bodies proximal to the outer cellular membrane of erythrocytes, thus the term *marginale*. This was the only form inducing disease within the United States until recently. Reports from other parts of the world, viz., Africa and Argentina, indicate that a subspecies, A. marginale var. centrale, is involved in pathogenesis. This second species has now been demonstrated in the United States.

Most authors refer to A. marginale as a protozoa-like microorganism, although recent investigations indicate a close relationship to rickettsial organisms.

TRANSMISSION

Transmission is accomplished by biologic and mechanical means. Biologic transmission involves arthropod vectors, especially the bloodsucking varieties. Of

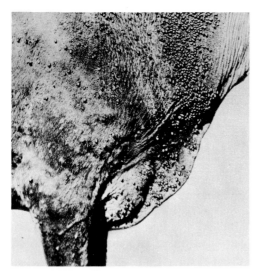

Fig. 10–1. Neck and shoulder of a bovine heavily infested with ticks, the vectors of anaplasmosis.

prime importance are the ticks (Fig. 10-1, Table 10-1), although mites, lice, mosquitoes, and biting flies also have been incriminated. These vectors feed on cattle harboring the disease and then on uninfected animals, thus transferring the pathogenic agent. A significant factor in this method is the interval between feedings. Experimental evidence indicates that the chelicera and other sucking mouth parts of the vector must be wet with blood to cause an active translocation of Anaplasma bodies. In most climatic areas, any disruption in feeding exceeding 4 minutes lowers the virulence of the agent because of coagulation of the erythrocytes. However, the ability of tick species to incorporate

the microorganisms within their bodies in a virulent state must not be discounted. It has been proved experimentally that female ticks can retain Anaplasma for as long as 6 months without lowered pathogenicity.

Research has disclosed the phenomenon of transovarian transfer of A. marginale from the maternal tick to the ova. The infective organism remains viable in the ovum and larval stages of the tick from one season to the next. In the instance of the three-host tick, the infective organism may be transmitted at any blood meal. This means of transmission is apparently the way Anaplasma can over-winter in an enzootic area. The developmental stages in the life cycle of arthropods will be discussed later.

Numerically, arthropods exhibit wide seasonal fluctuations. The most critical period involving population peaks of anaplasmosis vectors occurs during the months of late summer and early fall. Statistical field studies correlate the incidence of the disease with the variation in vector populations.

Mechanical transmission involves the transfer of blood from one animal to another via various operations performed on herds. Of prime concern are castration, dehorning, ear tagging, tattooing, vaccination, and blood sampling done with bleeding needles. Transmission normally occurs when sanitation has been neglected.

Transmission in utero has been reported in certain bovine species. Dams free of the

TABLE 10-1.　Principal Tick Vectors of Anaplasmosis in the United States.

Scientific name	Common name	Stages of life cycle when Anaplasma organism carried
Argas persicus	Fowl tick	Nymph, adult
Dermacentor variabilis	American dog tick	Larva, nymph, adult
Dermacentor andersoni	Rocky Mountain spotted fever tick	Egg, larva, nymph, adult
Dermacentor occidentalis	Pacific coast tick	Egg, larva, adult
Dermacentor albipictus	Winter tick	Larva, nymph, adult
Rhipicephalus sanguineus	Brown dog tick	Nymph, adult
Ixodes scapularis	Black-legged tick	Larva, nymph, adult

disease and then infected during gestation have produced calves carrying the pathogenic organism. However, this transfer mechanism is believed to occur infrequently. The animal is more likely to abort than to give birth to a full-term calf.

FACTORS INFLUENCING SUSCEPTIBILITY

All breeds of cattle and many other ruminants are susceptible to anaplasmosis. Worldwide surveys have demonstrated that the Anaplasma organism has a marked specificity toward ruminants, especially those of the bovine species. Therefore, anaplasmosis is principally considered as a disease of cattle.

Sheep and goats appear to demonstrate some degree of susceptibility; however, in most instances, the infection is a latent, mild type. In 1955, a breeding ewe flock grazing on wheat pasture in western Kansas was observed to have a "debilitating condition." The etiologic agent was isolated and classified as A. ovis.

A significant factor in epizootic areas is the ability of wildlife, especially native deer, to harbor the pathogenic organism. Known carriers in the United States are black-tailed deer, white-tailed deer, and mule deer of western range areas. In many instances deer do not succumb to the disease but serve as reservoirs, thus posing great danger as a potential source for infecting healthy beef and dairy herds through bloodsucking vectors.

Some Anaplasma-like organisms of an obscure nature have been isolated in swine and poultry, but to date, researchers have not elucidated the A. marginale relationships. Anaplasma-like infections in man have not been reported.

Three factors influencing susceptibility are of note: (1) age of the individual, (2) level of sanitation and health in the herd, and (3) the degree of parasite control.

The correlation of age and susceptibility has been substantiated by numerous research and field studies. Calves normally have an innate physiologic ability to resist the Anaplasma invasions and generally evidence a mild type of infection. Conversely, older animals do not resist infection by Anaplasma and readily succumb to the effects of the destruction of red blood cells. In some herds, mortality in animals over 1 year of age has exceeded 50%. Further, animals over 3 years of age may have a mortality of 90%.

Although sanitation and parasite control are not directly related to susceptibility, they nevertheless have an influence. Herds allowed to become heavily parasitized and cattle maintained in unsanitary environments demonstrate increased susceptibility.

CLINICAL SIGNS

Signs are primarily related to erythrocyte destruction and the resulting anemia. In mild infection, often seen in calves, the pulse rate quickens, diarrhea or constipation may be present, respiration increases, and temperature may range from 103 to 106°F. Some important field signs involve changes in behavior. Calves go off feed (anorexia), become "dumpy" or dejected, remain apart from the rest of the herd, and are exhausted because of anemia. In most instances, infection in young animals is short-lived, and they rarely succumb to anaplasmosis.

Signs in mature animals present a different picture. The rapid destruction of erythrocytes by the Anaplasma organism places great stress on the animal. The severity of the anemia is represented by extremely rapid or labored breathing; a pulse rate of 100 to 140; a temperature of 104 to 107°F; excessive salivation; general weakness and pallor; frequent urination; inappetence; psychotic, frequently aggressive, actions due to anoxia of the central nervous system; and abortions during all stages of pregnancy (chiefly caused by the high fever).

Icterus (jaundice) is commonly observed in cattle infected by the Anaplasma organism. Principally, it is caused by increased concentrations of bilirubin in the circulating plasma fluids. This results in a yellowing of epithelial tissue, especially mucous membranes of the muzzle, nasal cavity, and eye. Mammary-gland tissue is also discolored; consequently, anaplasmosis has often been termed "yellow-teat disease" by stockmen.

PATHOGENESIS

The incubation period occurs following transmission of the etiologic agent to a susceptible animal; a state of Anaplasma proliferation and dissemination develops in the new host. The interval is between initial exposure and microscopic detection of Anaplasma bodies on stained blood films, or the manifestation of clinical signs of the disease. The incubation period may last 15 to 45 days, depending on the resistance of the host and the virulence of the organism.

The clinical period is manifested by icterus and anemia with secondary signs. It is estimated that the parasite invades 50 to 77% of the circulating erythrocytes during this period. Hematologic changes involve a net decrease in erythrocyte numbers. Erythropoiesis, or red blood cell production, cannot meet the demands caused by the rapid invasion and destruction of blood cells. During this brief period, the animal lapses into an acute or peracute condition; death occurs rapidly. If, however, antibodies can be produced during this period, the animal will probably enter a period of convalescence. The Anaplasma apparently acts as foreign protein (antigen), thus causing antibody formation. In young animals, fetal splenic erythropoiesis, coupled with antibody production, accounts for suppression of the disease; removal of the spleen in calves results in exacerbation of all signs and death. In older animals, antibody production to combat Anaplasma is less efficient, and increased blood formation to replace damaged cells is more difficult to achieve.

If an animal survives a mild infection, or if clinical signs improve following treatment, the Anaplasma may have been destroyed or the organisms may be lying dormant in the spongy portions of the long bones. The animal is classified as a carrier when microscopic blood stains reveal a decrease in Anaplasma, anemia and icterus subside, and the organism is lying dormant in some part of the body. During this period, a delicate immunologic balance exists between host and parasite. Experimentally splenectomized bovine carriers lose this equilibrium and relapse into clinical states.

POSTMORTEM SIGNS

The gross postmortem findings are indicative of the stress imposed on the hematopoietic system during infection. Pallor and icterus of the tissues are evident. Erythropoietic suppression is shown by a watery consistency of the blood and a lighter red color. The spleen is greatly enlarged; the liver is also enlarged, with icterus and distension of the gallbladder.

DIAGNOSIS

Diagnosis is accomplished by observing clinical manifestations and employing laboratory tests. Infected animals exhibit anemia, icterus, rapid or labored breathing, temperature of 103 to 107°F, general weakness, irrational behavior, loss of appetite, constipation, and a decrease in milk production. Rapid death is common during the acute and peracute stages of infection. When anaplasmosis is suspected from outward signs, blood studies are necessary to verify a tentative diagnosis. When microscopic examinations of stained blood samples disclose Anaplasma bodies, diagnosis is confirmed (Fig. 10-2). However, these bodies rapidly deteriorate and, in many instances, are not observable under a microscope. Therefore, additional diagnostic methods may be necessary.

The main serologic techniques used to diagnose anaplasmosis are: (1) the comple-

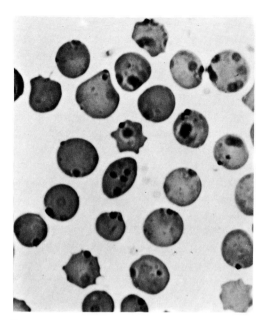

Fig. 10–2. Appearance of blood cells of a bovine infected with anaplasma marginale.

Maryland. It eliminates the delay involved in sending blood samples to laboratories for analysis. The test may be done at the farm or ranch, and the results are available within 10 minutes. One drop of colored antigen is mixed with one drop of serum separated out of a blood sample; macroscopic colored clumps indicate a positive reaction.

Because signs of anaplasmosis are similar to those of other bovine diseases, caution must be maintained during diagnosis. Anemia and jaundice are indicative of gastrointestinal poisoning, acute parasitism, hepatic malfunction, and eperythrozoonosis. High temperature and rapid or labored breathing are signs of pneumonia, shipping fever, blackleg, and leptospirosis. Rapid death is a prime indication of anthrax in cattle.

PREVENTION AND CONTROL

The methods used to prevent and control anaplasmosis vary in relation to the geographic distribution of the disease and its incidence. Northeastern and midwestern sections of the United States, where the incidence is low, may successfully prevent the disease by avoiding mechanical transmission during surgical procedures and control of the arthropod vectors. Known infected cattle in these areas can be isolated and given high dosages of tetracycline to clear them of the disease. Vaccination is not practiced when the potential incidence and threat of transmission is so limited. As a precaution, herds with a known infected animal can be tested to determine the presence of carriers. Those animals identified as carriers can be disposed of or treated and cleared.

The vaccine currently available is effective in developing sufficient resistance to prevent the clinical disease. However, even natural exposure of young calves does not eliminate the possibility of the carrier state.

In marginal areas of higher potential infection, such as parts of the Tennessee Val-

ment-fixation test, (2) the fluorescent-antibody technique, and (3) the antigen-antibody agglutination test.

The complement-fixation test is not only a valuable aid in diagnosing clinical cases, but also is 95% reliable in disclosing latent carriers. However, this method requires delicate procedures and is time-consuming.

The fluorescent-antibody technique subjects blood samples suspected of containing Anaplasma to fluorescein isothiocyanate. This precipitates an antigen-antibody-dye complex, which, under ultraviolet light, fluoresces a yellow-green, thus denoting infection.

The antigen-antibody agglutination test is extremely accurate in diagnosing the carrier state. It employs a capillary tube in which a mixture of serum and a prepared antigen is incubated for 24 hours. Macroscopic aggregates in the tube indicate an infected animal, whereas absence of the aggregates is evidence of a negative test.

A field test for anaplasmosis has been developed by scientists at the National Animal Disease Laboratory at Beltsville, ley, some herds can be kept free of losses by strict control of vectors and mechanical transmission and by constant screening for infected cattle. Herds controlled in this manner are susceptible to infection and to sick animals. Some herds in the same area are controlled by the owner's resignation to the suppression of clinical disease and his acceptance of a carrier status. This is either accomplished by vaccination or by feeding low levels of tetracycline during the vector season. Feeding an antibiotic, tetracycline, to lactating dairy cows must be done carefully to avoid residues in milk. Obviously, the dual approach to control in marginal areas creates management problems for owners trying to maintain disease-free but susceptible cattle.

Where the disease incidence is high, clinical disease is often avoided by not having susceptible cattle. Massive exposure is reduced by attempts to control vectors, but some managers purposely infect young calves with the blood of known carrier adults to provide protection against clinical disease. Other producers rely on vaccination to develop enough resistance to protect against severe clinical signs. The cattle in these herds are potential immune carriers.

TREATMENT

Cattle with even severe clinical signs of anaplasmosis can be restored to health. Tetracycline is effective in eliminating the organism. However, severely anemic animals are difficult to handle. The anxiety and excitement of loss of oxygen causes aggressiveness, and sufficient exertion can cause the animal to collapse and die from attempts at movement or restraint. Blood transfusions are required to sustain some animals during treatment. Frequently, the restraint required to administer blood is enough to cause death. Cattle have been known to charge handlers attempting to move them and to drop dead in the middle of the charge.

Less severely affected cattle can be successfully handled and treated. Some may even be medicated for mild signs by adding tetracycline to the feed. The dosage and duration of treatment determine whether the animal is cleared and susceptible or is cured of clinical disease but is still infected and a carrier.

Parasites—Internal and External

Livestock management is continuously challenged to control the effect of parasites. The job of achieving efficient production and maintaining healthy animals is difficult enough without the added disadvantage of feeding and nourishing a parasite population.

When an animal harbors a parasite that lives either in or on it, that animal is a host. Being a host is a generous status that productive livestock can ill afford. Parasites can be considered in two general categories. External parasites live on or are nourished by the outside of an animal. These are arthropods, such as lice, flies, fleas, ticks, and mites. Internal parasites are usually associated with the digestive system and are commonly considered as worms or a larval form of them. Examples of internal parasites are round worms (Fig. 10-3), tapeworms, flukes or nematodes, cestodes, and trematodes.

Parasites reproduce themselves and may live parts of their stages of life free in the environment or on other hosts. As a consequence, they are difficult to control, difficult to eradicate, and are constantly affecting the growth and health of animals. Internal parasites not only deprive the host of nourishment required to sustain the parasite but also damage the tissues they invade. Cattle infected with the medium stomach worm, Ostertagia ostertagi, become unthrifty and have poor

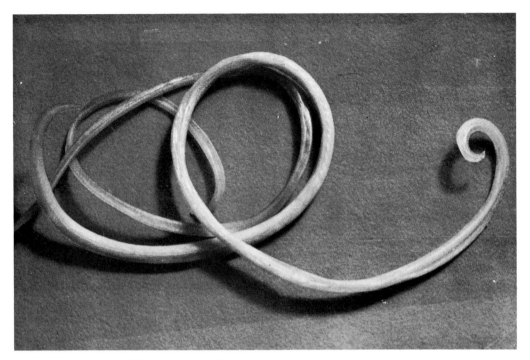

Fig. 10–3. General appearance of roundworm of livestock.

weight gain, watery diarrhea, rough hair coat, and so-called "bottle jaw" (Fig. 10-4). External parasites also nourish themselves at the expense of the host and cause sufficient discomfort and irritation to cause the host to expend and waste energy in nervous rubbing or efforts to relieve the irritation. In heavy infestations, Bovicola bovis (the biting or red louse of cattle) can cause significant loss of blood in the host. No relationship between parasite and host can be considered favorable to the host. In fact, most are decidedly detrimental.

Young animals are usually more severely affected by parasites than are older animals. This may be the result, in part, of development of resistance with age or may be a reflection of the relative numbers of parasites to the size of the body. Debilitated or poorly nourished animals are more severely affected because the host has less energy to share with the parasite.

How, then, can management plan and arrange to avoid losses caused by parasitism? As with the prevention of any infectious agent, one must first understand the way parasites live, the various animals used as hosts, and the environment most suitable for their survival. Such knowledge allows the possibility of interrupting the life cycle by creating unfavorable conditions before the parasite affects the host.

Fortunately, the science of parasitology has produced most of the knowledge required about the common parasites of domestic animals. Life cycles have been studied in detail. Both external and internal parasites, as well as the diagnostic signs produced by infection, have been described. This knowledge has resulted in control measures that can be applied to reduce the losses to livestock production.

LIFE CYCLES AND CONTROL MEASURES

It is not the purpose of this text to provide a detailed description of all common parasites and the appropriate control measures. Many excellent comprehensive texts are available, as well as up-to-date information in animal-science magazines, journals, and bulletins. Some examples are

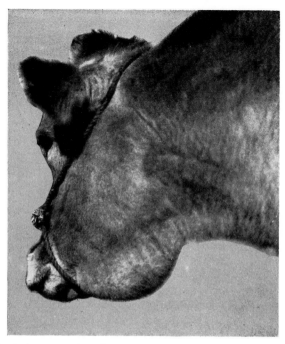

Fig. 10–4. "Bottle jaw" in the bovine resulting from parasitism. (From Gibbons, WJ: Clinical Diagnosis of Diseases of Large Animals. Philadelphia, Lea & Febiger, 1966.)

given, however, to illustrate the use of knowledge to formulate control measures.

Internal Parasites

Ostertagia Ostertagi

Ostertagia ostertagi, the medium stomach worm of cattle, is an economically significant parasite. The adults are found on the mucosa of the abomasum, where male and female mate and produce eggs. Eggs are passed out of the digestive tract in feces. Depending on the conditions of temperature and moisture, the eggs will hatch and larval stages will develop. Adverse weather during winter reduces the chances of survival of free living stages. Under ideal conditions, larvae reach the infective stage in 2 weeks or less. The infective stage could survive in soil or vegetation for several months. Cattle, as the host, ingest the infective stage along with vegetation. The larvae enter and live in the mucosa of the abomasum for a varying period. Infective larvae can develop into the adult stage in 3 weeks. However, this

development may be inhibited or delayed for as long as 6 months. This delay may be caused by the immunity of the host, but research indicates it is more likely caused by conditioning of the infective larval stage in a cold environment prior to ingestion.

Clinical signs of diarrhea and unthriftiness occur when the young adult parasites emerge from the gastric mucosa. At this time, there are considerable changes in the stomach wall, which becomes thickened and red around the white nodular areas where the adult emerged. The number of parasites determines the extent of damage and the severity of clinical signs.

This information suggests several possibilities for control. The first and most obvious is to deprive the free-living, infective stage of the larvae of a host for a sufficient time to prevent survival. This would require removing cattle from potentially infected pastures for several months, possibly over winter, and may not be economically feasible. The second possibility is to prevent the adult females from producing eggs to perpetuate the cycle. At present, the administration of drugs, such as thiabendazole and levamisole, to infected cattle destroys the adults. This relieves the host from the burden of supporting the parasites and reduces egg contamination. The larval stages remain embedded in the gastric mucosa and must be dealt with as they emerge. In severe infestations, administering antiparasitic drugs every 10 days eventually eliminates the supply of infective larvae.

Bots

The complete life cycle of Gasterophilus intestinalis, the bot fly, requires 1 year. In this instance, the parasite is a larval stage that attaches to an area of the stomach of horses. Although not considered the most serious parasite of horses, it does cause digestive disturbances and colic. Occasionally, the larvae may perforate the stomach wall, thereby causing a fatal peritonitis.

The cycle begins with the mating of adult flies, and females deposit eggs on the hairs of legs, body, neck, and throat of the horse for about 2 weeks. When the horse licks or bites the area where eggs are deposited, the first-stage larvae develop and penetrate oral tissues. After about 3 weeks of development, the larvae emerge and pass to the stomach as second-stage larvae. In 3 to 4 weeks of further development, third-stage larvae attach to the stomach wall and remain there for as long as 10 months. The third-stage larvae eventually detach and pass out in the feces to burrow beneath the surface of the ground. After pupating in the ground for 1 to 2 months, the adult fly emerges to repeat the cycle.

This cycle suggests several control measures. The first is to control the fly population and prevent the depositing of eggs. Pasture rotation and limitation of the number of animals on pastures help to reduce contamination. However, control of bot infection is most effective when horses are treated during the fly season to eliminate the second-stage larvae. Carbon disulfide is effective but highly toxic and should not be used on severely debilitated or pregnant mares. Organophosphorus drugs, dichlorvos and trichlorfon, are effective against migrating and attached bots.

Lungworms of Swine (Metastrongylus sp.)

The life cycle of swine lungworms is interesting because the earthworm is an intermediate host and is necessary for development of the larvae. The adult lungworms live in the bronchi and bronchioles of the lungs. Their presence in the lungs may cause inflammatory changes that are linked with pneumonia in young pigs. Even more significant is the potential association of the lungworm with swine influenza virus. The parasite is considered to cause sufficient damage or debilitation to require control measures. Eggs produced by the adult worms are coughed up in an embryonated stage, swallowed, and eliminated in feces. Certain species of earthworms ingest the embryonated eggs, which then develop into first-stage larvae. These larvae penetrate the esophagus of the earthworm, move into the circulation, and lodge in the earthworm's heart. Then, larvae undergo several molts to the third stage in about 2 weeks. There are reports of viable larvae remaining in the earthworm for as long as 4 months. In fact, eggs have reportedly survived in pastures before ingestion by earthworms for as long as a year or more. Eggs usually survive only several weeks on the surface of exposed ground, but survive for a longer duration if buried in feces to a depth of 1 foot or more.

When ingested by pigs, the earthworm is digested, and the infective larvae are released. The larvae then penetrate the intestinal wall and are assumed to follow lymph channels to lymph glands or to enter the circulation, migrating to the right side of the heart or lungs. The larvae develop during this migration so that, on arrival in the air passages of the lungs, they are adults that are ready to reproduce. The migratory time in the definitive host from ingestion of earthworms to passage of embryonated eggs is approximately 3 weeks.

The life cycle of swine lungworms suggests several methods of control.

1. If pastures that are not conducive to earthworm populations are chosen, the necessary intermediate host is reduced.

2. If contaminated pastures are devoid of swine for a month, the embryonated eggs on the surface will be destroyed by sunlight.

3. If pigs are prevented from rooting by nose rings, the ingestion of earthworms will be reduced.

4. If pigs are raised in confinement on concrete, the earthworm host is almost eliminated.

5. If pigs are treated with drugs to destroy adult lungworms, the cycle is broken. There are several drugs reported effective. Levamisole is considered highly effective and can be administered in feed or water.

External Parasites

Psoroptic Mange of Sheep (Sheep Scab or Scabies)

This disease has been economically significant and debilitating to sheep. The USDA and State Departments of Agriculture have sponsored research and eradication programs to the end that it is virtually nonexistent in the United States today. The mange mites, Psoroptes ovis, live on the hindquarters, sides, and shoulders of sheep. By burrowing into the skin and feeding, they produce intense itching and a lymph-and-serum-encrusted lesion. Infected sheep rub, bite, and kick at the affected area, thus denuding the area of wool. The disease can progress and cause death (Fig. 10-5).

The life cycle of the mite is short (about 3 weeks) and is completed entirely on sheep as the host. The female and male adults

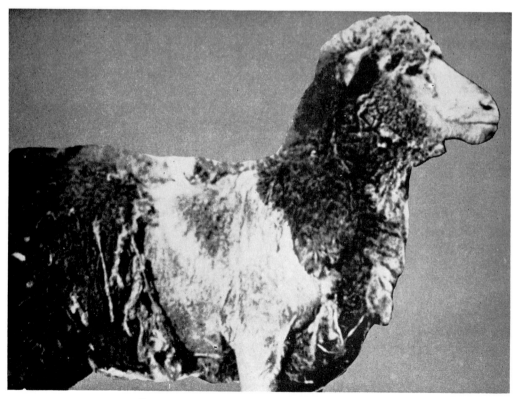

Fig. 10–5. Psoroptic mange. Note denuding of wool.

feed on the skin of the host. The female lays her eggs on the edge of the lesion on the skin. Tiny, six-legged larvae emerge from the egg and develop into eight-legged nymphs and then into eight-legged adults. Adults are 0.6 to 0.8 mm in length and can be seen if scraped from the edges of the lesion. The mite is host specific and does not survive for long when not on the host. Transfer from animal to animal is by direct contact.

The life cycle, which is completed on the host, gives no alternative for control. The mite must be killed while on the host. Because of the cycle, the mite cannot exist in any form in the environment except on an infected sheep. Since there are no intermediate hosts or larval forms to perpetuate the mite other than on the animal, eradication is more possible. Methods used include dipping or spraying with 0.5% toxaphene and preventing movement of infected sheep.

DIAGNOSIS OF PARASITISM

Such clinical signs as debilitation, progressive loss of weight, intermandibular edema or "bottle jaw," anemia, diarrhea, loss of hair coat or wool, itching, rubbing, or skin lesions are characteristic of many diseases. Such general signs should alert the diagnostician to the possibility of a parasitic disease. Confirmation of parasitic disease must be made by finding direct evidence of the presence of parasites in or on the animal in sufficient numbers to cause disease.

The evidence required for confirming the existence of internal parasites is usually available in the feces in the form of eggs or larvae or adult stages. There are various laboratory techniques and methods for recovering eggs and larval forms from feces. Adults may be grossly visible. Forms of external parasites may be seen in the form of eggs attached to hairs, or the adult mite or louse may be seen on the skin. Microscopic forms may be scraped from the edges of lesions caused by external parasites.

Effective control of any parasite depends on measures to interrupt its life cycle. To interrupt life cycles that have variable characteristics, one must identify the parasite. A diagnosis of parasitism is not complete without identifying the specific parasite involved.

As noted in the examples cited, control measures are adapted not only to the life cycle of the parasite but also to the susceptibility of forms of the parasite to various drugs. There are two critical considerations for using drugs to rid animals of parasites:

1. The drug used must be tolerated by the host at the level or dose required.

2. The drug must not leave residues in the animal that could be toxic or harmful to people if the animal is to be used for food production.

In general, insecticides, anthelmintics, or any drugs used to rid an animal of parasites have been thoroughly investigated. Safe, effective dosages have been calculated, and containers are labeled to indicate these dosages as well as potential adverse reactions and contraindications for the use of the drug. In addition, drugs approved for use in or on food-producing animals have specific, published restrictions regarding their use to prevent harmful residues in either meat or milk.

CHAPTER 11

Diseases Characterized by Tumors

These are three forms of tumors of farm animals. Leukosis and cancer eye are quite common; melanoma is not. Until the cause of the various forms of malignant growth is understood, prevention and control are not possible. Research to understand cancer in farm animals not only is significant for efficient production of food but, more important, is the contribution to prevention and control of cancer in human beings.

RECOMMENDED READING

Theilen, GH, and Madewell, BR: Veterinary Cancer Medicine. Philadelphia, Lea & Febiger, 1979.

Bovine Leukosis, Cancer Eye, and Melanoma

BOVINE LEUKOSIS

Cattle, as well as other species used for production of food, do not have a high incidence of diseases characterized by tumors or neoplasms. Of the neoplastic diseases of cattle, bovine leukosis is the most common. The term, bovine leukosis, refers to a group of four clinical diseases: (1) juvenile or calf leukosis, (2) thymic leukosis, (3) skin leukosis, and (4) adult enzootic leukosis. The most common and most significant of these is adult enzootic leukosis.

All four forms of bovine leukosis are associated with tumor formation. Calf or juvenile leukosis may cause tumors from birth until 2 years of age. All lymph nodes are usually involved and are noticeably enlarged. The thymic form occurs in cattle approximately 2 years of age, and the tumor is a large mass extending from the chest along the neck to the throat. The cutaneous form appears as scattered wart-like growths on the skin of cattle from 1 to 3 years of age. Enzootic adult leukosis usually involves the lymph nodes, abomasum, heart base, uterus, and other areas, such as the postorbital and spinal canal. The occurrence of lymphosarcoma (the name commonly used for the tumor formation) is sufficient to have caused significant economic loss from death or condemnation of slaughtered carcasses. The incidence throughout the world varies, but some European countries have attempted eradication programs because of the potential economic loss. In 1977, the rate of condemnation of adult cattle with lymphosarcoma by USDA inspection was 21/100,000.

Signs and Diagnosis

The lesions are easily observed if well developed. External lymph nodes, such as those under the jaw (mandibular nodes), in front of the shoulder (prescapular), in the fold of the flank (subiliac, Fig. 11-1), and above the mammary gland (supra-mammary or superficial inguinal, Fig. 11-2) become noticeably enlarged. All or only one or two nodes may be enlarged. Palpation of lymph nodes by the rectum is also an aid to diagnosis.

Enlarged lymph nodes in either the juvenile or adult form, the swelling along the neck in the thymic form, and the characteristic lesions of the skin in cutaneous form are not completely diagnostic without some confirmation by microscopic examination of the tumor tissue. A variety of signs may be produced by tumors growing in the abomasum, base of the heart, and uterus. When any of these organs is involved without noticeable lymph node swelling, diagnosis is more difficult. Although there is occasional spontaneous regression of tumors, the disease usually progresses to fatal termination.

Cause

The cause of the disease is not completely understood. There is conclusive evidence of the association of a viral infection with enzootic adult leukosis and the cutaneous form. This virus, called the bovine

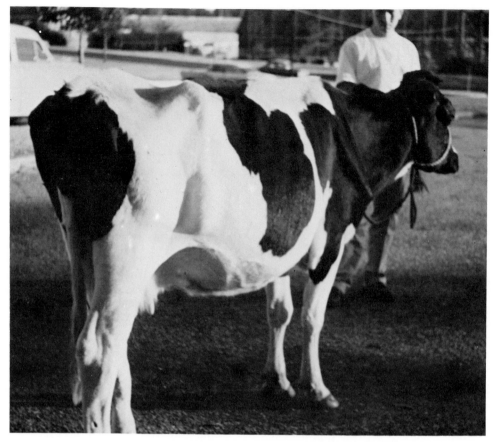

Fig. 11–1. Enlarged subiliac lymph node caused by bovine leukosis.

leukosis virus (BLV), and/or antibodies to the virus have been demonstrated from all cattle with the adult form. However, bovine leukosis virus has also been recovered from cattle with no signs of disease. Further, antibodies to the virus have been detected in a fairly high percentage of the U.S. cattle population. Estimates from various surveys indicate that more than 15% of all cattle are infected with the bovine leukosis virus. A higher percentage of dairy cattle than beef cattle is infected.

Other factors, such as environmental, genetic, and immunologic, may be involved in the development of adult bovine leukosis. Investigations in progress may help to clarify the cause of bovine leukosis as well as other neoplastic diseases.

Transmission

The determination of an infectious agent in association with bovine leukosis has stimulated investigation of transmission. Other species can be experimentally infected with BLV, but only bovine are known to be naturally infected. Vertical transmission has been suspected for many years because of a relatively high incidence of disease in some closed herds. Calves born to infected dams have antibodies to BLV before ingestion of colostrum. This indicates transplacental infection. Also, virus particles in the milk of infected cows cause infection in susceptible calves. Experimentally, blood from infected cattle inoculated into uninfected cattle causes infection.

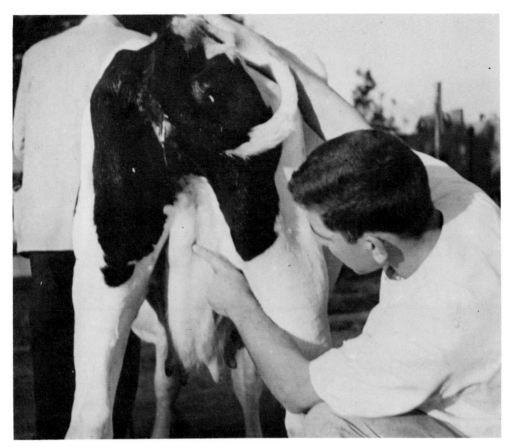

Fig. 11–2. Enlarged superficial inguinal lymph node caused by bovine leukosis.

This reportedly has been accomplished by intradermal injection of a minute amount of blood containing as few as 2500 lymphocytes. As a result, the possible transmission of the infection by biting insects, as well as by hypodermic needles and other instruments used on cattle, is under investigation. The possibility of secretions or excretions from infected cattle with virus-carrying leukocytes also presents potential transmission by direct or indirect contact.

The possibilities for infection with bovine leukosis virus seem numerous. The fact that the virus has infected a large proportion of the cattle population is confirmed by surveys determining the presence of antibodies in herds in various parts of the United States. However, infection with BLV does not always result in tumors or clinical disease. In fact, most infections are not accompanied by any clinical signs. No evidence indicates loss of production as a result of infection unless tumors or neoplastic tissue occur. There are estimates that less than 1 of every infected 1000 cows develops the clinical disease.

Prevention and Control

Three factors are helpful in designing a plan for preventing or controlling a disease. The first is a means of accurate diagnosis. The second is the precise cause of the disease. The third is the method of transmission. Applied to bovine leukosis, only parts of all three factors are well understood.

The bovine leukosis virus is closely associated with enzootic adult leukosis. Other influences on the cause are not clear. Knowing the potential of the virus is at least a starting point. When the virus is not present, there is no disease. Prevention must stop the virus from infecting susceptible animals. The virus can be present in cattle without any evidence of disease. Animals carrying the virus must be kept apart from noninfected or susceptible animals to prevent transmission. Therefore, a means of detecting the virus in the apparently healthy animal is necessary.

The means to detect the presence of the virus by diagnostic tests are available. At least antibodies to the virus can be detected. This would indicate infection. Several tests can accomplish this. The AGID (agar gel immuno diffusion) test is perhaps the most easily conducted. A negative result to an antibody test would be good evidence of no infection. If animals with negative test results are prevented from contact with infected animals, their secretions and excretions, and potential vectors, the disease can be prevented.

Keeping uninfected animals free from the vectors requires more knowledge. There is good reason to believe that biting insects feeding on the blood of an infected animal could subsequently inoculate other animals by transferring virus-carrying lymphocytes when biting. Until the identity and capabilities of all potential vectors are known, control will be difficult.

Control and prevention consist of identifying infected cattle, keeping noninfected cattle separated from infected cattle, and removing infected cattle from the herd. If new cattle are to be added to the herd, their negative status must be assured by several tests before they can come in contact with uninfected animals.

There are ongoing investigations to determine answers to questions about this disease. The following general information is of interest:

1. The bovine leukosis virus is not known to cause disease in other species.

2. There is no evidence to indicate transmission of BLV by artificial insemination.

3. The BLV, although eliminated in milk from healthy cows, is destroyed by pasteurization.

4. Vigorous and thorough surveys of persons in close contact with cattle infected with BLV have shown that there is no indication of human infection by BLV.

CANCER EYE OF CATTLE
(Squamous Cell Carcinoma)

Cancer eye is a relatively common neoplastic disease of cattle. The cancerous growth is found most often on the eyelids (Fig. 11-3). It may start as a benign-appearing papule and may grow slowly to a large, raw mass that destroys the normal skin and adjacent structures, invade the surrounding and deeper tissue, and be transferred to other locations in the body by the circulating blood. As the tumor grows, the raw surface becomes infected by bacteria that increase the normal tissue destruction. The eye itself is usually destroyed if the carcinoma is allowed to progress. All breeds of cattle are susceptible, but the disease occurs most commonly in Hereford or white-faced breeds. Although the eye and eyelids are the primary location, the area of the vulva is another site of growth.

The disease is of economic significance. If allowed to progress unchecked, it could eventually cause death. Many animals are salvaged by premature marketing, and those showing extension of the cancer are condemned for slaughter.

The cause of the disease is not completely understood. A viral agent is suspected. Carcinogenic irritants, such as wind, dust, and sunlight, are considered possible contributors. Some consideration is given to the possibility of genetic predisposition. None of these causes has been proved.

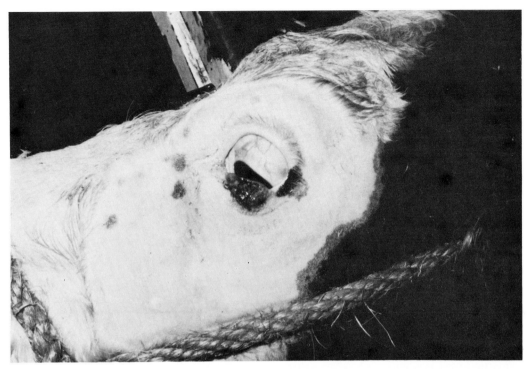

Fig. 11–3. Cancerous eye of cattle.

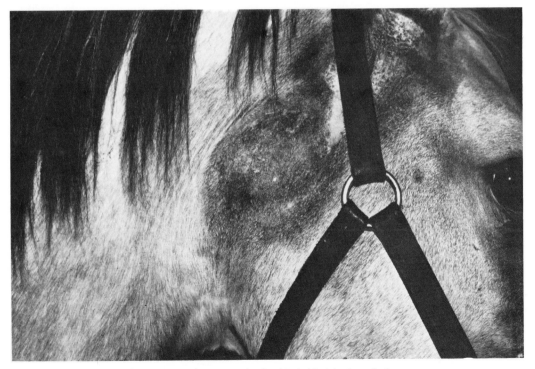

Fig. 11–4. Melanoma under the skin behind the jaw of a horse.

Without knowing the specific causes of this type of cancer, prevention is not possible.

The disease can be controlled or retarded in the individual animal by surgical excision of the growth in the early stages. If this is done when the growth is 1 to 2 cm, disfiguration when healed is minimal and usefulness is not impaired. Even if the growth has progressed to the point where removal of the eye is necessary, the life and usefulness of the animal are prolonged significantly. However, when the growth has metastasized to the lymphatic system, it cannot be arrested. Other means of destroying the growth successfully are implantation of radioactive gold, excision by cautery, and freezing.

MELANOMA

Melanomas are most often found on old gray horses (Fig. 11-4). These tumors are pigmented and usually are located under the skin at the base of the tail. Although also found on dark-skinned cattle, they are considered benign for cattle. The disease is classed as malignant in horses and spreads throughout the body. Early excision is the best control, but is less likely to be successful for horses (Fig. 11-5). Although pigmented skin is a factor in the cause of melanomas, there is no known means of their prevention. Although rarely observed, malignant melanomas have been reported on sheep and goats.

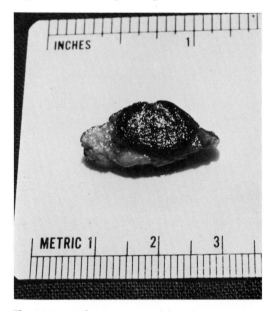

Fig. 11–5. Melanoma removed from horse in Figure 11–4.

Index

Page numbers in italics indicate figures; those followed by "t" indicate tables.